Mind Museums

Mind Museums offer a fresh perspective on the heritage of mental health, bringing museums into sharp focus. Drawing on interdisciplinary approaches from architecture, museum and exhibition design, and heritage and museum studies, it examines former psychiatric asylums that have been converted into museums.

The book presents a comprehensive investigation of mind museums, the first of its kind in Europe, and explores their potential in raising awareness and dismantling the stigma surrounding mental health. Through an in-depth examination of selected European examples, Lanz describes what mind museums are and how they came to be. The innovative visitor studies carried out at the *Museo di Storia della Psichiatria* in Reggio Emilia, which are presented here, explore people's encounters with mind museums and reveal the profound impact of such experiences. By uncovering the power of these heritage sites in facilitating discussions on mental health, civility, and care, Lanz provides new insights into the emotive capacity of the museum and visitors' reflexivity at place-based memory sites.

Mind Museums will be of great interest to scholars and postgraduate-level students engaged in the study of museums, heritage, exhibition design, architecture, and mental health. It should also be of interest to heritage professionals, particularly those working in mind museums and other similar sites, such as prison museums and sites of conscience.

Francesca Lanz is an assistant professor of interior architecture at Northumbria University, Newcastle upon Tyne, UK. Her research combines different disciplinary approaches, theories, and practices from architectural, museum, and critical heritage studies, focusing on the role of the built environment and museums in contemporary societies, with a particular emphasis on neglected heritages and challenging memories.

Museums in Focus
Series Editor: Kylie Message
Australian National University, Australia

THEDISOBEDIENTMUSEUM
@REBELMUSE_ROUTLEDGE

Committed to the articulation of big, even risky ideas, in small format publications, 'Museums in Focus' challenges authors and readers to experiment with, innovate, and press museums and the intellectual frameworks through which we view these. It offers a platform for approaches that radically rethink the relationships between cultural and intellectual dissent and crisis and debates about museums, politics, and the broader public sphere.

'Museums in Focus' is motivated by the intellectual hypothesis that museums are not innately 'useful', 'safe' or even 'public' places, and that recalibrating our thinking about them might benefit from adopting a more radical and oppositional form of logic and approach. Examining this problem requires a level of comfort with (or at least tolerance of) the idea of crisis, dissent, protest, and radical thinking, and authors might benefit from considering how cultural and intellectual crisis, regeneration, and anxiety have been dealt with in other disciplines and contexts.

The following list includes only the most recent titles to publish within the series. A list of the full catalogue of titles is available at: https://www.routledge.com/Museums-in-Focus/book-series/MIF

Museum Representations of Motherhood and the Maternal
Mother Stuff
Rebecca Louise-Clarke

Mind Museums
Former Asylums and the Heritage of Mental Health
Francesca Lanz

⌐MUSEUMS IN FOCUS⌐

Logo by James Verdon (2017)

Mind Museums
Former Asylums and the
Heritage of Mental Health

Francesca Lanz

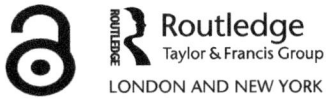

Routledge
Taylor & Francis Group
LONDON AND NEW YORK

First published 2024
by Routledge
4 Park Square, Milton Park, Abingdon, Oxon OX14 4RN

and by Routledge
605 Third Avenue, New York, NY 10158

Routledge is an imprint of the Taylor & Francis Group, an informa business

British Library Cataloguing-in-Publication Data
A catalogue record for this book is available from the British Library

ISBN: 978-1-032-19398-4 (hbk)
ISBN: 978-1-032-19399-1 (pbk)
ISBN: 978-1-003-25897-1 (ebk)

DOI: 10.4324/9781003258971

Typeset in Times New Roman
by MPS Limited, Dehradun

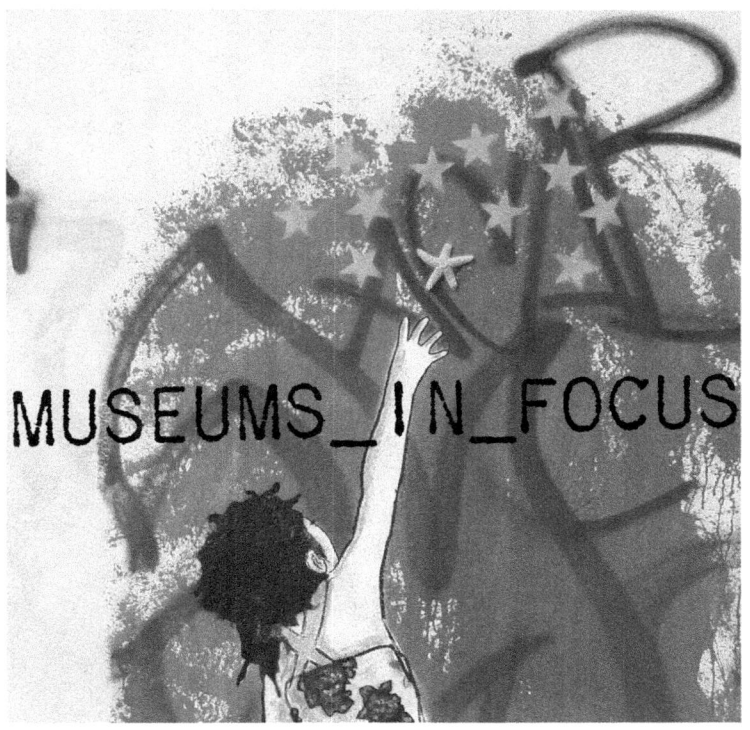

Anonymous graffiti, Athens. Image and logo by James Verdon (2017).

For Miki
[in loving memory of mum]

Contents

Acknowledgment[1]

Writing this book involved a lot of translating. It required the translation of methodological approaches and theoretical frameworks from one discipline to another and back again. It involved the translation of concepts, ideas, and ways of thinking from one language to another, but also within different cultural and social contexts, and within diverse academic contexts. The process of translation extended to hours of video interviews and implicated not only translating from Italian to English, but also trying to capture and translate a greatly visual and intensely emotional way of communicating made of gestures, pauses, and meaningful silences, into written words. It also involved the translation of a large corpus of new knowledge acquired through three years of research and fieldwork into this short but long-windedly worked-on book. Translation always implies a great deal of interpretation. It involves appropriation and re-writing, demanding research, and an understanding of the originating context as well as comprehension of the destination.

I would like to take this opportunity to express my gratitude to every individual who has contributed to this process over the years. From family and friends who supported me with their love and day-by-day help, to the many passionate guides and curators who generously spent days and hours with me, taking me around their museums, exchanging emails, and sharing documents and thoughts. I am also thankful to all the people I met and spoke with on-site during my visits, workshops, and interviews, and to the numerous brilliant scholars, researchers, and museum professionals I had the fortune to come across during these three years, for their invaluable support and advice. In particular, I would like to acknowledge the support provided to me by my hosting institution, the School of Arts and Cultures at Newcastle University. I am deeply grateful to Prof. Rhiannon Mason for welcoming me in the School; all the colleagues at the Department of Media Culture Heritage, for making me feel part of a vibrant research community; the School and University research staff support and, in particular, Kerry Dodds for their precious help; and above all, Prof. Christopher Whitehead, for his supporting and inspiring mentorship. I extend my heartfelt thanks to Bruce Davenport for his invaluable assistance with the editing and language polishing. His work has gone far beyond mere proofreading and has made a significant contribution to this project. Finally, I would like to sincerely thank the members of the network *Mente in Rete*, and Pompeo Martelli (*Museo Laboratorio della Mente*), Teresa Melorio (*MAPP – Museo d'Arte Paolo Pini*), Alice Ceppatelli and Alessandro Massi (*Manicomio di Volterra*), Luigi Armiato (*San Servolo Museum*) and Stella Mann (*GHM – Glenside Hospital Museum*), for the invaluable support they offered to my study. I owe a particular debt of honor to Chiara Bombardieri, director of the *Biblioteca Scientifica Carlo Livi* and chieft curator of the *Museo di Storia della Psichiatria*, Francesca Poli, Lucia Romoli and Erica Casini, the guides of the *Museo di Storia della Psichiatria* in Reggio Emilia, Georgia Catoni, from the *Musei Civici di Reggio Emilia*, and Giorgia Lombardini, architect at the Reggio Emilia municipal technical office, for their assistance and openness towards helping me out during my study. Without their support, a significant part of the research beyond this book would not have been possible. Lastly, but most importantly, I want to express my deepest gratitude to the many research participants who contributed to my study. They generously shared with me not only their time but also their private memories, intimate thoughts, and emotions, which enriched and shaped this work in profound ways.

As in any translation, I am aware that something may have been lost in the process, but hopefully something has been gained as well. I hope my perspective and interpretation have been able to add nuances that were previously absent in the debate. Above all, I wish for this book to inspire others to research how we can approach mental health through its heritage, and how this heritage can support debate and aid in dismantling stigma and promoting awareness about 'madness'.

Note

1 This book ensues from the research project ReMIND, *Reactivating Neglected Heritages, Reweaving Unspoken Memories: A Study on the Adaptive Reuse of Former Asylums into 'Mind Museums'*. ReMIND received funding from the European Union's Horizon 2020 research and innovation programme under the Marie Skłodowska-Curie grant agreement No. 841174. It was carried out by Dr. Francesca Lanz at Media, Culture, Heritage in the School of Arts and Cultures, Newcastle University, from June 2019 to May 2022.

Introduction

This book is grounded in the belief that there is a need to talk more about mental health from the perspective of both historical and current issues and practices. This is what Catharine Coleborne, internationally renowned scholar in the field of mad studies and histories of mental health and psychiatry, also maintains in her most recent book *Why Talk About Madness* (2020). Here, Coleborne advocates for the need 'to imagine new ways of thinking about madness' (3) and suggests that 'talking about madness is possible through the archives of institutions, personal stories, the spaces and places of confinement and living histories of these, through exhibition, artworks and through advocacy and community support' (Coleborne 2020: 53), alias what we could refer to as *the heritage of mental health*. In this book, I explore how 'talking about madness' can be done through such heritage, in museums; more precisely in a specific type of museum, which I call 'mind museums'. Mind museums are museums hosted in the disused spaces of a former mental asylum whose display focuses on the history of their premise, and on past and contemporary approaches to the care and treatment of mental health. However, a mind museum is not solely a museum of social history or a museum of the history of psychiatry, nor is it simply a former asylum building restored and conserved as a museum of itself. Rather, it is a site-specific and place-based cultural institution whose work taps into the material and immaterial heritage it conserves and exhibits, with the ultimate goal of promoting awareness and dismantling the stigma and stereotypes surrounding mental health today.

It is my assertion here, that there is such a thing as the heritage of mental health and that such heritage, although being currently largely neglected and overlooked, holds great potential to offer new and engaging ways to talk and think about mental health. This book focuses on this heritage, bringing museums into sharp focus, with the intent to encourage increased research engagement with mental health and its heritage, especially within critical heritage and museums studies. Whilst there is a growing corpus of

DOI: 10.4324/9781003258971-1

studies focusing on the history of 19th-century mental asylums and their afterlife, with contributions from various academic disciplines notably including history, geography and architecture (in particular: Ajroldi et al. 2013; Calabria 2020; Calabria et al. 2021; Franklin 2002a; 2002b; Gibbeson 2020; Moon et al. 2015; Osborne 2003; Topp et al. 2007), little has been said about former asylums as heritage and their memorialisation. On the other hand, while research into the so-called 'mad studies' has flourished in recent decades (Coleborne 2020: 2, 73–75), few studies have specifically addressed museums and other forms of public display concerning the heritage of mental health.[1] This book fills this gap.

In this book, I will define mind museums, positing them within the contemporary landscape of the heritage of mental health. Here, not only will I describe what mind museums are and how they came to be, but I aim to provide an understanding of what they do and with which effects, with key regard to their potential for unlocking productive discourses around mental health, civility and care. Virtually every scholarly work that focused on museums and exhibitions about mental health has speculated on the potential key role these may have in promoting the construction of new knowledge about mental health, with beneficial effects on public awareness about it and its care (in particular, see: Coleborne 2020; Rodéhn 2020; Armiato and Martelli 2019; Dudley 2017; Moon et al. 2015: 70-85; Barnes 2014; Pascarelli 2013; Coleborne and MacKinnon 2011; Flis and Wright 2011; Labrum 2011; Brüggemann and Schmid-Krebs 2007). However, none of them – with the exception of the work by Lachlan Dudley (2017; 2018) and Cecilia Rodéhn (2020) – goes further in probing such assumptions through any kind of in-depth field work-based study. Furthermore, thus far, the vast majority of the studies focusing on museums and mental health, and especially those seeking to evaluate their impact, have focused on the therapeutic or well-being benefits of museum visits with key regard to people with lived experience and service users (e.g. Barnes 2014; Dondici 2009; Chatterjee & Noble 2013; Silverman 2002) and have disregarded these museums' effects on general visitors. My work draws on and expands these studies by delving into these overlooked questions with the aim of providing new evidence-based, critical insights into the social role of mind museums and the heritage of mental health.

This book builds upon a three-year-long research project on the reuse and musealisation of former asylums funded by the European Union with a Marie Skłodowska-Curie individual fellowship in 2019. Key questions at the core of the study revolved around the relationship existing at mind museums between each site's materiality, its associated memories and the overall museum project, meaning its spaces, display and practices. How are the material and immaterial features of the building (re)used at these museums and with which intents and effects? What is the potential of mind museums for effecting attitudinal change in visitors that may help to dismantle stigma and promote collective responsibilities of care? The research aimed to explore such questions developing at the intersection between museum and heritage studies, architecture, and museography.

The distinction between what in Italy is called *museografia*, and what in the anglosphere is termed 'museums studies' and the implications of such a transdisciplinary approach may elude most of the readers who are not familiar with both traditions. Emblematically, there is no English term for the Italian *museografia* – commonly and awkwardly translated in an anglicised version as museography. Likewise, there is no effective way of translating 'museum studies' into Italian. However, this is not a merely linguistic issue, but rather a matter of different, often disconnected, approaches to and traditions in the study of museums that results in different methodological and theoretical ways of thinking about museums and analysing their displays and design (Lanz and Leveratto 2023; Tzortzi 2015; Mason et al. 2018a). To avoid opening up a long digression on the roots and outcomes of such different approaches that falls beyond the scope of this introduction, it will suffice to say that while museum studies are mainly concerned with curatorial aspects of a museum project and its display, to analyse their contribution to the museum's meaning-making with chief regard to its political and cultural context and possible social effects; a museographic approach instead delves into such questions by primarily focusing on the architectural project of a museum and the design of an exhibition, to explore their aesthetic and epistemological implications.

My approach involved the mingling of these different but complementary disciplinary perspectives and research methodologies to develop a nuanced investigation of mind museums, the first such study in Europe, the understanding of which has been fundamentally aided by such a transdisciplinary analysis. This approach also meant that a particular emphasis was placed on mind museums' exhibitionary environments, meaning the physical built and experiential spaces of the museums. This is in no way to suggest that the museum environment and its contents can or should be considered separate or distinct, since I firmly believe the opposite. However, reflecting an emerging line of thought within critical display analysis that accounts for the key role of the museum environment in museums meaning-making (e.g. Whitehead 2016a; Whitehead 2016b; Tzortzi 2015; Moser 2010; Lindauer 2006), the role of mind museums' spatial contexts has been given primary consideration when assessing what mind museums are and can be.

Previous studies have already articulated the evocative or 'atmospheric' 'power of the place' in relation to memory sites and commemorative events (Sumartojo and Graves 2018; Sumartojo Shanti and Sarah Pink 2018; Sumartojo 2016; Edensor and Sumartojo 2015) and sites of conscience[2] (Ševčenko 2010; Ševčenko 2011). Similarly, recent scholarly work has largely recognised that – because the museum experience has a key sensory, non-discursive dimension that produces embodied and affective forms of knowledge in response to the material, aesthetic and spatial qualities of the exhibition – the museum environment plays an important role in how visitors make meaning out of such experiences (Smith 2021; Sumartojo 2019; Smiths et al. 2018; Watson 2015; Witcomb 2012). Drawing on that, my working hypothesis was that former asylum historical complexes and their remnants have specific attributes and characteristics that not only make these places historically and socially meaningful but also, and crucially, able to 'speak' about mental health. What I was interested in understanding was whether such evocative nature of this heritage, including but not limited to the 'atmosphere' of its places, does provoke strong emotional and empathic reactions in visitors, and if these, in turn, can support and contribute to reflection that 'cannot exist [...] if reason is not associated with an emotion' (Drugman 1998).

With Sharon Macdonald, I here assume that the built environment and 'physical entities, such as buildings and landscapes' do have agency and 'capacities' that 'inevitably shape how those entities are experienced, related to, and acted upon' (Macdonald 2006: 106; Macdonald 2009; Dovey 1999; Miller 2005; Gieryn 2002). As Macdonald highlighted, to assess this agency while discussing heritage is not only pertinent but paramount, even more so when the heritage in question was originally expressly designed and realised to have some specific effects. 'What or how building and environments mean or do' – Macdonald says – 'are questions of considerable importance for heritage and public memory' (2009: 25). This book investigates these questions by focusing on the case of mind museums, former asylums and the heritage of mental health and asking if and how the heritage of mental health and its public presentation and representation can help dismantle old stereotypical definitions to produce new and more progressive understandings about madness.

The volume is organised into three main chapters. Building on existing literature, the first chapter surveys the broader issue of asylums' rise to their fall, and reuse. It outlines the asylum's development across Europe between the end of the 18th and the middle of the 20th century; it considers the phenomena of their disuse and abandonment and the hurdles faced in reusing neglected and stigmatised built heritage. The overarching objective of this chapter is not to offer an historical account of asylums' development across Europe. Rather, its aim is to provide an understanding of the extreme complexity of the built heritage of the asylum today, forasmuch as the asylum 'both holds "madness" within its walls and helps produce representations and definitions of madness that travel beyond these walls' (Coleborne and MacKinnon 2003: 1). This idea is central to the last section of the chapter titled 'Palimpsest', which presents a personal account of a visit to an abandoned asylum in

Tuscany and concludes the historical overview offered by the chapter by introducing questions pertaining to the chances and challenges surrounding asylums and their traces, including material remnants as well as the meanings and memories encapsulated in these heritage sites.

The second chapter focuses on the residues and remnants left behind by asylums after their closure to discuss how these 'traces' (Anderson 2021) coalesce, sometimes coexisting and sometimes conflicting, into the contemporary landscape of the heritage of mental health. This chapter defines in outline mind museums by tracing their origins within 19th-century asylum collecting practices, positing their birth as asylum museums within the deinstitutionalisation movement, and eventually discussing their more recent developments into contemporary institutions aimed at promoting awareness about mental health in the past and the present. To do that, it equally draws upon a comprehensive literature review on the subject, and a comparative study of the main mind museums in Europe, with an in-depth focus on Italy. When it comes to the politics of mental health and the landscape of mental health heritage, the Italian context is both unique and paradigmatic. Italy, in fact, not only fully embraced and further developed ideas and approaches promoted by the anti-psychiatric movement that was thriving in 1950s across Europe, but it is the country that more than any other, pushed forward the deinstitutionalisation process up to closing all the mental hospitals of any kind, including forensic ones (Donnelly 1992). Mental health treatments in Italy today are solely administered on a voluntary basis; mental health care is fundamentally community-based and informed by social psychology and radical psychiatry ideas and approaches as they were developed within the Italian movement *Psichiatria Democratica* under the leadership of the influential psychiatrist Franco Basaglia (Babini 2011; Foot 2014). In Italy, since the closure of all asylums, several research projects have been promoted aimed at studying and conserving the heritage of mental health, which in turn have spurred a number of different initiatives for the valorisation of that heritage and promoting public engagement with it. As a result, today in Italy, there are numerous mental health collections and various cultural institutions, including several museums, whose work revolves around the heritage of mental health. Several of those have recently spontaneously grouped together to create a network for the valorisation of the heritage of mental health, called *Mente in Rete*.[3]

The final chapter of this book focuses on one of these museums, the *Museo di Storia della Psichiatria* in Reggio Emilia (Italy), and unfolds around the discussion of this single case study to answer some of the key questions addressed in this book pertaining to the relationship at mind museums between the site materiality, its associated memories and the overall museum project, and their combined role in determining visitors museum experience and its effects.[4] The findings of this study suggests that visitors' encounters with the heritage of mental health at mind museums not only enable them to draw connections between past and present stories of mental health, but ignite curiosity, elicit memories and spur emotional responses and empathic reactions. Such connections often happen at a very personal and affective level and eventually facilitate introspective reflections, producing extremely enduring memories and prompting proactive responses to the visit experience.

Delving into the case of mind museums and the Reggio Emilia museum, in particular, allows me to explore intertwined questions of the cultural and architectural project for the former asylums and other similar place-based memory sites, with key regard to mind museums' emotive capacity and visitors' own experiences and reflexivity. As I elsewhere articulated with Whitehead, while discussing exhibitions about migration (2020), an idealised proposition can be (and often is) made here, which is that visitors' encounters with certain kinds of museums and exhibitions may trigger empathetic responses based on the imaginative capacity to 'step into the shoes' of another person 'to understand their feelings and perspectives' (Krznaric 2016: x).[5] This, in turn – still ideally – may conduct visitors towards critical and ethical reflections on 'wicked' social problems and towards personal, collective and elective responsibilities of care. As we said there, besides problematising this assumption by taking into account visitors' foreknowledge and expectations, 'we must also problematise the further effects of the process. What does the reflection "do"? Does it lead to action on the part of the visitor to try to make the world a better place? What is that action? Or does it merely play out from an empathetic response with no particular concrete effects?' (Whitehead and Lanz 2020: 188). Such questions on the social power of museums resonate strongly in the final chapter and the conclusions of this book. In particular, I stress how mind museums and the heritage of mental health they conserve and exhibit are in effect able to productively 'unsettle' those who encounter them. Sharon Macdonald has called this the 'palimpsest effect' (2009: 191) to emphasise the potential of these heritage sites to 'allow different layers of the past to appear, variably, through their later accretions, and in so doing to disturb, prod, and raise questions – that is, to unsettle' and in that to offer a unique space for contemporary critique. Andrea Witcomb also speaks of the power of 'unsettlement' while discussing exhibition dealing with difficult histories (2012). Here, Witcomb also advocates for further studies that aim to explore audience engagement and responses to such kind of exhibitions that openly attempt to challenge visitors and invite them to 'rethink who they think they are and who they think they are viewing' (*ibid.*, 256): it is this book's ambition to contribute towards that.

Notes

1 Among them, the work by Catharine Coleborne stands out (Coleborne 2001; Coleborne and MacKinnon 2003; Coleborne and MacKinnon 2011; Coleborne 2020). Notably, the volume *Exhibiting Madness in Museums,* co-edited with Dolly MacKinnon (Coleborne and MacKinnon 2011), focuses on psychiatric collections and their display, with key attention given to Australia, New Zealand, Canada and the United Kingdom. The essays collected in the volume explore how histories and stories of psychiatry are remembered in and through exhibitions with the aim of producing knowledge about mental health today. Coleborne and MacKinnon's book constitutes one of the core references in my own work. However, with the sole exception of the essay of Nathan Flis and David Wright (2011), museums and built heritage of mental health are not directly explored within the publication.

2 The origins of the idea of site of conscience trace back to post–Second World War period, but the concept has only been properly developed since the 1990s and eventually strengthened and refined by the establishment of the *International Coalition of Sites of Conscience* (ICSC) in 1999. The Coalition was created with the aim to set out a network of institutions variously operating in the field of historic preservation, heritage and memory, which have committed themselves to promote, through their work, awareness, dialogue and citizen engagement on issues of human rights and social justice (Lloyd and Steele 2022; Ševčenko 2011; Ševčenko 2010). Since its establishment, the Coalition has grown considerably across the globe, today counting over 300 members in 65 countries and a wide array of cultural institutions chiefly including place-based museums, heritage and memory sites located at places of difficult, traumatic and painful past events. Following ICSC's own definition, what distinguishes sites of conscience is their commitment to act as 'safe place to remember'. Their overarching mission is to contribute to a better and more just future by preventing and counteracting forgetting and erasures in the belief that promoting dialogue and awareness can foster reconciliation and avoid repetition. Sites of conscience aim to encourage people not only to remember but to 'turn memory into action'. To that aim, they promote programmes designed to stimulate dialogue on pressing contemporary issues and human rights and fostering public involvement through their sites, seen as a 'bridge to connect past to present'.

3 *Mente in Rete* website: https://menteinrete.it/ [Last Accessed, March 2023].

4 Fieldwork was mostly carried out during the COVID-19 outbreak, deploying a 'methods assemblage' (Law 2004) that resorted to different visual and ethnographical methodologies, revised and adapted to account for both for my study's transdisciplinary approach and the challenging context within which it was carried out. This is further discussed in the following methodological note.

5 For a brief literature review, see Mason et al. (2018a) and Boyd and Hughes (2020) Chapter 2 'Exhibiting with Emotion', and Cecile Rodéhn (2020).

1 [Former] Asylums

Madhouses, lunatic asylums, mental hospitals: although, *contra* Foucault (1961), it did not happen within a sudden and systematic endeavour of mass internment and 'great confinement', since the 18th century different kinds of institutions and places specifically devoted and built for ministering to those considered 'mad' started to emerge across Europe. It was the dawn of the asylum, a 19th-century social and medical institution and an architectural place conceived and constructed in the wake of the positivistic psychiatric revolution of the time, in the belief that insanity should be treated and could be cured and that the built environment could play a role in doing so (Ajroldi et al. 2013; Jay 2016; Philo 2004; Piddock 2007; Topp et al. 2007; Yanni 2007). Throughout the 19th century, asylums developed and increasingly spread across the Western world, to become madness's 'natural place' and its 'homeland' (Foucault 1961 (2006): 47, 386). In the span of a century, they were born and then entered a relentless decline, which would eventually pave the way to their end and which still largely defines them in the popular imaginary.

Although the birth of the asylum was an international phenomenon, inasmuch as Foucault himself defined and discussed it as a European phenomenon (1961 (2006): 52), and whilst comparisons and analogies can be drawn between the history of asylums' evolution in Europe and overseas, there have been many variations between these institutions across time and within different cultural, geographical and socio-political contexts. There were, in fact, remarkable differences, even at a local level, in the regimes, social and medical approaches, as well as specific spatial solutions, put into place for the purpose of the management of people suffering from mental health issues. Thus asylums, despite their similarities, should not and cannot be in any account regarded as all being the same. That being so, this chapter outlines the development of the asylum in Western Europe from its inception at the turn of the 19th century to its end in the second half of the 20th century. In this chapter I will discuss the birth and evolution of the asylum in

DOI: 10.4324/9781003258971-2

relation to the progresses, evolutions, revolutions and U-turns of medical and socio-cultural approaches to 'madness' through time, with special attention given to how this was reflected in the built fabric of psychiatric institutions. To do that, I draw on a growing corpus of studies on asylum history mainly undertaken within the fields of medical history, geography, architectural history and cultural sociology. Most of these works have been developed in the Anglosphere (especially the United Kingdom, United States and Australia) and they concentrate on the establishment and growth of mental health care institutions in these countries, in relation to the important medical bodies and legislative changes inaugurated during the period from the mid-19th century to the 1960s.[1] The overarching objective of this first part of the book, however, is not to offer a historical account of asylums' development across Europe, but rather to provide an understanding of the extreme complexity of the built heritage of the asylum today, forasmuch as the asylum 'both holds "madness" within its walls and helps produce *representations* and *definitions* of madness that travel beyond these walls' (Coleborne and MacKinnon 2003: 1, italic added). This book focuses on how these representations can help dismantle old stereotypical definitions to produce new and more progressive understandings about madness today.

The asylum before the asylum

'The Victorian age' – says Andrew Scull – 'saw the transformation of the madhouse into the asylum into the mental hospital; of the mad-doctor into the alienist into the psychiatrist; and of the madman into the mental patient. And while it would be a grave error to confuse semantics with reality, it equally will not do to treat these verbal changes as no more than a succession of euphemisms masking a fundamentally static reality' (Scull 1981: 6). Indeed, although there is a historical continuity of a sort linking the birth of the asylum with other places and practices in place in medieval times which were devoted to the treatment of those considered as insane, as Scull himself suggests the asylum is a 19th-century institution and invention, and, at first, it was a significant social and medical innovation.

Before the establishment of the asylum, there was no systematic approach or facility chiefly devoted to the treatment of madness and in no country before 1800 was medical supervision a legal requirement in provision for the insane, nor was there warranty of good care (Philo 2004; Scull 2011: 105–108). Even less was there any place specifically designed, purposely built and solely devoted to host, cure and contain mad people: insanity was mainly a family responsibility, as much as a burden and a shame. Many of those 'mentally disturbed' were looked after – and hidden – as best their family could within the domestic walls. Some could retire, more or less willingly, at informal pseudo-religious sites of 'holy water' resorting to hermit-saint, shrines and other blessed remains as means of cure combined, at best, with medications based on long-established humoral medical theories. Others were sheltered together with the poor, the elderly and the sick in monasteries, local parishes or *lazarettos* (isolation hospitals) that offered 'hospitality' with no medical care implied. The majority, however, were just left 'wandering', begging for food and shelter, broadly rejected by society and mostly tolerated or simply ignored as long as they were not troublesome, in which case they were locked up. An exception to this is the town of Geel in the Flanders, which since the 13th century up to the present day welcomed and hosted people with mental disorders. The story tells that St Dymphna, an Irish princess, hid in Geel to escape her father, who was driven mad by the grief of the loss of his wife and claimed her in marriage. Dymphna became revered as the Saint protecting those suffering with mental health problems and a sanctuary was erected in the centre of the mediaeval town of Geel. This became a place of pilgrimage, but also a place where many of those who were not cured by the saint's holy power were eventually abandoned. A cloister was built to host them, but that soon proved inadequate; local residents thus started to take in those who needed shelter in exchange for help at work and on the fields. Geel, however, remained a rare instance of care in the community.

During the 17th century, those among the population who were more marginal and socially disrupting, such as those considered dissolute and the idle, often including the pauper and the 'lunatic', were detained in different kinds of facilities, none of which, however, were purposely built or run for the sole and specific purpose of ministering to the 'mad'. These mainly included houses of corrections, prisons, workhouses and paupers' hospitals. Some eventually specialised, more incidentally than on purpose, in dealing with the mentally ill – such as the Bethlem hospital in London, one of the eldest and possibly most (in)famous asylums in the United Kingdom and beyond (Andrews et al. 1998; Jay 2016; Philo 2004). Much like Geel, the origins of the Bethlehem hospital are also traced back to the 13th century and to a religion-based myth. The story goes that a London alderman, named Simon FitzMary, upon returning to his home country from the Crusades and spurred by a mystic experience he had in the Holy Land, erected a priory dedicated to St Mary of Bethlehem on his own land in Bishopgate. As with other hospitals of the time, the priory worked as a shelter, offering hospitality and support to those in need, including the pauper, the elderly, the ill and those at the fringe of society, among which were a good share of mentally troubled people who soon became the most numerous population. From here unravels the long story of the Bethlem asylum, from a cloister to a modern, contemporary mental hospital.

Alternatively, a minority of those struggling with their mental health were treated in informal and pragmatic arrangements, mainly private institutions, operating for profit in what was later emblematically termed the 'trade in lunacy'. Rarely located in purpose-built structures, these institutions were usually hosted in adapted buildings offering a private service, mainly for better-off 'mad-men' and 'mad-women' who were put under the oversight of the 'mad doctor' who ran the business. Known in England as madhouses and in France as *petit maisons*, these arrangements were mainly private institutions in some cases managed by a charitable organisation. Madhouses were at first limited in number, but they continued to grow over the course of the 18th century. Madhouses varied in quality. Whilst historical studies point out how madhouses have also been a 'forcing-house for the development of psychiatry as an art and science' (Porter 2002: 100; Scull 1981), and although some could be supportive places of care, most madhouses were wretched places characterised by corruption and cruelty, where those ministering to the patients largely resorted to physical restraints – including chains, harness, enclosures beds and other kinds of fetters – corporal punishments and terror therapies, in a regime of fear and coercion and terrible abuses. At that time, these conditions were, sadly, prevalent in many of the places hosting people with mental health problems of different kinds.

In 1814, the British philanthropist Edward Wakefield denounced the case of James Norris, an inmate at the Bethlem hospital, whom he found in a deplorable state during a visit to the asylum. Wakefield's exposure of Norris's condition, and the campaign he initiated for the improvement of the provision for the insane across the country, contributed to the formation of the Committee on Madhouses in 1815 (First Report from the Committee on the State of Madhouses 1815), which ultimately led to the first reform in the county asylum law in the United Kingdom. In those years, similar scandals surfaced in other institutions in other countries with similar effects. The same happened in Italy, too, albeit with some delay compared to other countries. In 1902, an investigation carried out across several madhouses in the northeast of the country, reported terrible mistreatment of the inmates found by the inspectors in gruesome medical and hygienic conditions. The San Servolo male asylum in Venice was one of the worst cases – reported for the horrific status of the people hosted in its premises, who were kept in chains, neglected and physically and sexually abused for years. The asylum was run by the Catholic religious order known in Italy as *Fate Bene Fratelli*, alias the Brothers Hospitallers of Saint John of God, under the supervision of a superintendent mad-doctor, the monk Camillo Minoretti. The report on the San Servolo asylum became a national scandal. The public indignation and the political shame for having allowed that to happen paved the way for the first Italian national legislation on the provision of those considered mentally ill, the so-called *Legge Giolitti*, dated 1904. The law established for the first time the criteria for interment, which included being 'socially dangerous' and 'publicly embarrassing' because of 'socially inappropriate behaviours' and introduced the mandatory requirement to have a forensic ward in any mental asylum. The law would be updated several times over the following decades, but it remained substantially unchanged, grounding Italian mental health treatment legislation until the ratification of the so-called *Legge Basaglia* in 1978 (Babini 2011).

These scandals on the one hand, spurred the very first medical and legal reform of psychiatric care across Western countries that would set the ground for the rise and development of asylums. On the other hand, their denunciation and exposure, which was largely visual, started to create a visual imaginary of these places as grim, noxious and tainted places. This image persisted and grew in the following centuries passing on from madhouses, to asylum and then to psychiatric hospitals. The paintings *Yard with Lunatics* (1793–1794) and *The Madhouse* (1812–1819) by Francisco Goya, inspired by his visit to the Zaragoza madhouse, or the widely reproduced painting *The Rake in Bedlam* (1734) by the English artist William Hogarth, are emblematic of the visual transliteration of madhouse spaces into an artistic trope. From this moment on, the asylum would become a recurrent theme in different artistic and cultural productions, from painting to poetry, from novel to recent film productions (Rondinone 2019), contributing to the formation of a collective imaginary of the places devoted to ministry to the insane in which madhouses, asylums and mental hospitals tend to all blur together as one single grim space of desperation.

The origins and harbingers of asylums are to be found in that context, at the end of the 18th century and in the early decades of the 19th century, when a new approach to the treatment of the insane, the so-called moral approach, started to find its way across medical knowledge and practices within Western European countries and overseas. The development of the 'moral approach' and the subsequent advent of the asylum should be therefore understood thus as an evolution as much as a reaction against and a key departure from approaches and provisions for the treatment of the insane in the 18th century's enlightened despotism. Driven by a philanthropic ardour, more humanist in its intention and inherently moral in its therapeutic approach, this new approach led to a wide lunacy reform that eventually culminated in the invention of the asylum – the first purpose-built facility for the care of the 'mad' (Babini 2011; Scull 2011; Porter 2002; Scull 1981). The legendary story of the French alienist Philippe Pinel (1745–1826), setting inmates free from chains at Bicêtre in 1793 and Salpêtrière in 1795, has become a 'myth-like' symbol of this new course of action and established Pinel as a sort of founding-father of the moral approach and the asylum.[2] Figureheads of this 'revolution' were European alienists and philanthropists, who were active between the end of the 18th and the early years of 19th century,[3] whose ideas and pioneering experiences were taken up in the second half of the 19th century by a second generation of psychiatrists, thinkers and reformers across Europe and overseas who implemented these ideas and practices further, and helped to consolidate them: it was the dawn of the asylum.

Driven by a positivistic optimism, champions of the moral approach sought a more humanist and rational basis for the care and treatment of mental illness. They believed that insanity could be cured, the patient could be re-educated and trained to decor and self-restraint and eventually returned to reason and reintroduced into society. This approach hinged on a more intimate and kind relationship between the treating doctor and patient, using a system of rewards and punishments, and the creation of an overall therapeutic and curative environment. Unlike the treatments offered in earlier regimes, which were based on the prevailing doctrine of humours, the moral approach was based on a meticulous classification and observation of the inmates, the establishment of types of disorder and behaviours which, in turn, informed the care of the patient and the administration of targeted medical treatments. As it aimed at exhorting patients to self-control, it tended to minimise forms of mechanical restraints and physical coercion and rejected earlier terror-based and fetter-reliant treatments, regarded as the symbol of previous unscientific, ineffective and inhumane approaches. The use of mechanical restraints, such as manacles and muzzles, was therefore steadily phased out, replaced by solitary confinement, soft restraint kits and the straitjacket – most of which are still in use today in hospital psychiatric wards. Every aspect of the overall therapeutic environment was considered and designed to support doctors' and nurses' everyday work and contribute to the cure and the management of patients. Talking sessions, therapeutic treatments, daily routines, physical exercise and physiotherapy, as well as religious and pastoral support were offered to patients. Different forms of treatments were constantly experimented with and implemented: from hydrotherapy to early forms of ergotherapy, art, music and movement therapy. Recreational activities, such as reading, painting, writing and playing games, were promoted as important elements of treatment that would help to divert and heal patients' minds. In all that, the built environment was believed to have a chief role.

The turn end of the 19th century saw the establishment of psychiatry as a medical science and the birth of the first professional associations, forums and scientific journals specifically devoted to psychiatry, such as the *Association of American Institutions* in 1884 in the United States (later *American Psychiatric Association*) and the Italian *Rivista*

Sperimentale di Freniatria in 1875, some of which are still up and running today. A series of laws were also ratified in most Western countries, where the moral approach spread, enacting country-wide legislations regulating and centralising the provision for the management of the insane; this crucially involved the implementation of national systems and the construction of networks of new purposely built facilities.

Unique buildings

Given the absence of any buildings designed specifically to house and assist people suffering with mental illness and given the practical implications of the moral approach, it was clear that a new kind of building was needed, and it needed to be invented. This happened through unrealised architectural projects, theoretical speculation and pioneering experimentation that led to the development of what Susanne Piddock calls 'the ideal asylum' – i.e. the idea of how an asylum should be, as theorised by doctors and psychiatrists (2007: 50–76; 2013).

The planning and design of the asylum became the object of attention and debate equally within the architectural and the medical spheres. Significantly, the first detailed treatises about how the asylum should be designed and run were written by psychiatrists. Jean-Étienne Dominique Esquirol (1772–1840), the favourite student of Pinel in France, wrote at length not only on new medical treatment for the care and cure of insanity but also describing how the asylum should be organised and designed to achieve that. He developed the asylum architectural typology of the *carré isolé* (single isolated blocks each of which housed a different function of the asylum), which would greatly influence asylums design within and beyond France. The Guislain asylum in Ghent (1857), the first Belgian asylum following the principles of the moral approach, was designed by Dr Joseph Guislain (1797–1860) and inspired by Esquirol's model. Dr Guislain was himself a physician from a family of architects with a chief interest in new medical approaches as much as in the design of their provision and his hospice set the standard for asylum architecture in Belgium during the second half of the 19th century and the beginning of the 20th century (Deblon 2017). In the United States, the psychiatrist Dorotea Dix (1802–2887) was a key figure in the establishment of first-generation asylums in North America, mostly designed following the so-called Kirkbride architectural model. Samuel Tuke, the grandson of William Tuke, founder of the York Retreat, in 1813 published a *Description of the Retreat*, which became a key text in the spread of moral treatment and its corresponding architectural approach. John Conolly (1794–1866), who pioneered a total non-restraint approach in the care and management of the insane (Conolly 1856), also wrote a very detailed treatise dictating best practices for the construction of county asylums (Conolly 1847). His ideas on non-restraint, despite initial reservations, were eventually embraced by several other psychiatrists across Europe influencing their practices as well as their approach to the design and management of psychiatric spaces. These included the Italians Carlo Livi (1823–1919) and Augusto Tamburini (1848–1934) at the Reggio Emilia asylum, and Luigi Scabia (1900–1934) at Volterra asylum in Italy.

On the other hand, the design of the asylum soon became a topic of discussion also in architectural symposia and specialist magazines. As one might expect, the realisation of such great buildings and major public infrastructure attracted considerable attention from architects of the time who were eager to implement their designs, not least to make their mark in architectural history. Furthermore, it required studies and experimentation from landscape to the interior design scale, offering a rare and considerable opportunity for typological and architectural innovation (see, in particular: Ajroldi et al. 2013; Piddock 2007; Yanni 2007). In effect, the design of each asylum happened within an unprecedented and never-again-repeated close collaboration between designers and doctors: insomuch that in many cases current historical architectural research has difficulty in ascribing the authorship of specific design choices to either the asylum designer or its superintendent doctor (McLaughlan 2015).

The first asylums to be designed and built were somewhat tentative and mostly drew on existing architectural types of other institutional confinement and healthcare facilities, such as the workhouse, the prison and the hospital; among these some – a few of which had been actually realised – deployed a Benthamite panopticon model.[4] However, they soon evolved into a totally new typology with several variations shaped around the needs of the moral approach and influenced by specific local building regulations and traditions, local legislations and about mental healthcare provisions as well as the specific treatment regime applied in each institution, and the vision of their superintended doctor. As noted by Catherine Coleborne, this variety of architectural models, may be considered as a proof of a search for an appropriate environment able to support therapeutic practices and it may reflect how the asylum, at least at its inception, was an institution focused on patients' wellbeing, care and treatment (2020: 45). Within the moral approach, the built asylum not merely was the place where medical treatments were to be administered to those suffering from mental illness, but it was one of its 'major weapons (perhaps the major weapon) in the struggle to cure the insane' (Scull 1981: 9). Research done within mad studies, geography and architectural histories of asylums has discussed how the asylums as built places had been important 'formative factors in changing modes of care [...] and in evolving forms of clinical research for the medical profession' (Topp et al. 2007: 1). However, notwithstanding the apparent centrality of care in the design of these buildings, social control and containment of the people in the asylum informed the overall architectural project of each asylum, its spatial arrangements and the design and decor of its interiors and outdoor spaces as much as medical considerations. Because of that, not only were asylums unique buildings in their functional programme and associated architectural typology, but also for the complexity and conflicting nature of this dual function and how this reflected on their design.

Neither solely a hospital nor merely a prison, hygiene and efficiency were key elements in the design of the asylum as well as security and surveillance. First, this is evident in their location. Their location in city's outskirts reflected the four main curative themes that emerge from early 19th-century treatises discussing asylum design and functioning such as those written by Tuke and Conolly, namely: 'proximity to society, access to nature, creating a tranquil environment (where individual treatment could be delivered), and disguising confinement' (McLaughlan 2015: 187). It was, in fact, recommended that asylums should be located in amenable and healthy contexts. An elevated site providing a visual connection to nearby conurbations was believed to be useful in reinforcing a patient's will to get better and return into society. The optimal site should offer good water provision, proper ventilation and convenient light exposure. It also should provided plenty of space to accommodate the several facilities needed for the asylum to function, including open-air spaces for patients' outdoor activities and cultivable soil to be used in ergotherapy and food provision, as well as space for possible future extensions. However, it would be naive not to recognise that the choice for building many asylums in rural settings and semi-rural settlements was dictated by such medical reasons and building best practices as much as by the will to socially and physically distance those who were considered 'insane', potentially dangerous and disruptive.

The double medical and social rationale of the asylum is also evident in their spatial layout and architectural design. Asylums' architectural complexes were usually physically marked by containment walls with a few controlled access points. These walls enclosed a self-sufficient microcosmos, comprising a variety of different spaces and buildings each of which was conceived and designed around principles of order and efficiency. Several spatial layouts have been implemented in time to guarantee security and control as well as hygiene and salubrity, and to support the daily management of patients within a therapeutic environment. The single building block typology was in time replaced by other more complex architectural models designed with regard to the site's orographic features, natural lighting and main wind direction, in order to accommodate the increasing variety of activities, treatments and patients to be hosted within its walls and reflecting patient's meticulous classification and their separation per gender, social rank, diagnosis and behaviours and to ease everyday activities, facilitate circulation across the buildings and shore up the staff's work. The most common ones, such as the cottage plan and the pavilion plan, consisted of a few central blocks and several surrounding detached buildings or pavilions. For security and practical reasons, buildings were usually one or two storeys high, variously disposed in the site following different planimetric layout – mostly grid or radial – and connected by enclosed corridors, galleries and large tree-lined avenues. Each pavilion was meant to host a different function from those strictly medical-related – such as infirmaries, staff residences, medical studies and treatment rooms – to a myriad of complementary facilities. Patients' wards were organised by function and by inmates' gender, diagnosis and social and detention status, and usually included dormitories, bathrooms and toilets, canteens, isolation rooms and punishment cells. There were also workshops (such as woodworking, typographic, shoe making, etc.), art and music rooms, halls, conservatories and galleries for social activities, administration buildings, libraries and archives. Other complementary structures were also built within the asylum estate and could include a mill, a bakery and kitchens, a chapel, a morgue, laundries, storage rooms, a graveyard and much more. Asylum complexes also included several open-air spaces and courtyards for outdoor exercise, vegetable gardens, cultivable fields, farms and stables. Originally small in scale, asylums soon started growing in size, becoming in many cases extremely large complexes and more like microtowns and self-sufficient colonies.

Equally important was the 'look and feel' of the asylum. The appearance and decoration of asylums' architectural complexes was in fact regarded as of equal importance for the creation of a curative environment as much as for a matter of representation. The asylum was more than a medical space, but also a major public work and built-in manifesto of a new scientific and political approach to the management of the medical and social problem of mental illness. Asylums thus were not only large complexes but also magnificent buildings. Outdoor spaces and gardens were objects of great attention. They showcased fountains, ponds, flowerbeds, trees and plants of different species as they were the main representation spaces towards visitors and inspectors, but also therapeutic spaces where the patients could walk, sunbathe, exercise and get engaged in gardening activities. The buildings' façades, especially those of the main buildings and those of the pavilions devoted to high-ranking (paying) patients, were splendidly decorated and carefully designed, often with references to palaces and countryside villas, showing architectural orders and polished wrought-iron balustrades and gates.

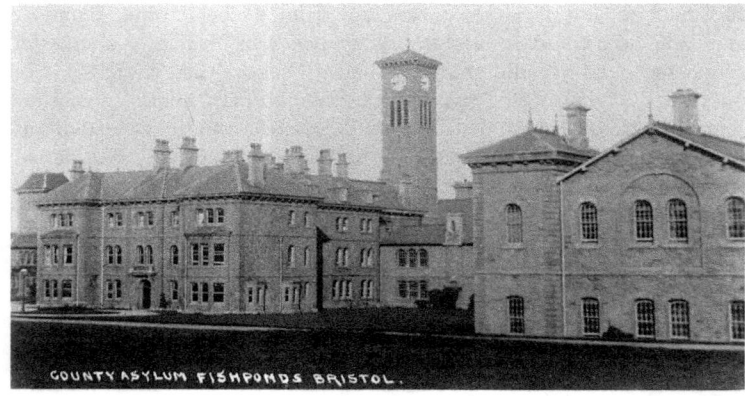

Image 1.1 Postcard of Bristol County Asylum in Fishpond, opened in 1861.
The Bristol Lunatic Asylum was approved as an asylum in 1857, following a more than ten-year controversy between the Bristol local authorities and the Commissioners on Lunacy, following the 1845 Mental Asylum Health Act, which imposed on Bristol authority to provide appropriate treatment and facilities for the mentally ill population, replacing those provisioned at St Peter's Hospital, a workhouse set up in a converted Jacobean house near St Peter's church in Bristol city centre. A competition was held for the design of the new Bristol Lunatic Asylum: out of the 27 proposals submitted, 3 were awarded prizes, and the 'neat but not gaudy' project by Thomas Royce Lysaght of Bristol was eventually selected for construction. Building works started in 1858 and the asylum finally opened in February 1861 (Davis n.d.; Smith 2017). Former Glenside Hospital today is the Glenside Campus of the University of West of England (UWE), hosting the faculty of Health and Applied Sciences since 1996. A museum of the asylum is hosted in the former asylum chapel.

The interiors of halls and galleries in administration buildings and those of major importance were also elegantly decorated with plaster-works, paintings and refined finishing equal to those of many major urban buildings. The general style of most of the other buildings of the complex and their interior design was inspired by domestic architecture and they were designed and decorated to be purposely agreeable with the intention of evoking in patients' memories a home-like and familiar environment that was believed to be beneficial for their tranquillity. Interior spaces were usually large and airy with high ceilings and numerous wide windows which created well-lit, ventilated and more hygienic spaces. Well-placed windows also allowed patients to view the surrounding landscapes, something that was believed to have a calming effect, supporting their self-restraint.

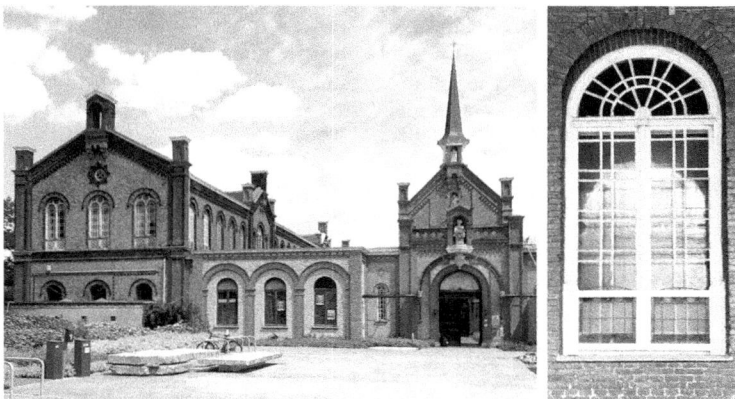

Image 1.2 The former Guislain asylum in Ghent (1857), photo of the main entrance and window detail.
In asylums, window bars and metal grids, when possible and often in common spaces, were avoided, and ingenious architectural solutions were implemented to make them less overtly visible and visually present. At the Guislain asylum, Dr Guislain designed a wood panel, reinforced with metal bars and decorated with stained glasses, which was secured on the low part of the window outfacing. This allowed the window to be open for ventilation, and the view to be free from visual barriers, but impeded patients from climbing over the windowsill and out. The Guislain asylum in Ghent today hosts the *Dr Guislain Museum*. Photos by Francesca Lanz, June 2022.

The interior space design was also meant to ease surveillance and patients' supervision and guarantee order. Rooms were of medium size, simple and straight shape with no blind spots. The furniture in patients' and common rooms was disposed along walls and in a single line to allow nurses and attendants to watch everyone in the space without visual barriers. Furniture was meant to resemble domestic environment; it was simple, sturdy and easy to clean. Wherever possible, both indoor and outdoor, fixed furniture was preferred over stand-alone and movable items. This was both for reasons of security, to prevent it being thrown in moments of outburst, and for control over the space layout and its uses. Interior finishing and materials were also a matter of careful design, dictated by cost, ease of maintenance, hygiene and security. Stone and brick were used as the main construction materials for fire prevention. In interior spaces, right angles were avoided, and room edges were often rounded to avert accidental injuries; pastel and white colours were commonly used for room decoration, and the use of washable painting was preferred over tiles, especially in patients' rooms.

Tiles, like other sharp materials such as mirrors, were mostly avoided for security reasons; equally, forks and knifes were not available to patients, who ate using soft pewter spoons. Shoes and clothes provided to patients as part of their uniform did not have laces, because they could be used as weapons against other patients or nurses or for self-harming.

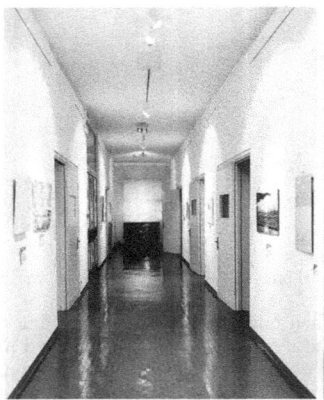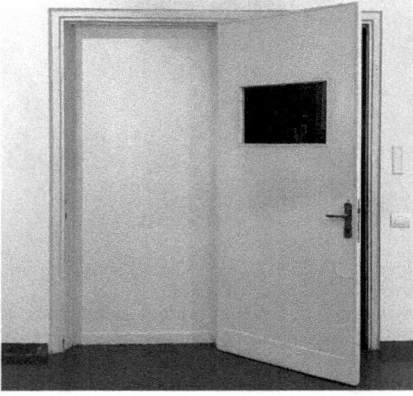

Image 1.3 The former Paolo Pini psychiatric hospital in Milan (date), interiors of the pavilion no. 7, former patients' ward and new venue of the MAPP – *Museo d'Arte Paolo Pini [Paolo Pini Art Museum]*.
The corridor has a simple brown ceramic tile floor and plastered white painted walls; room doors feature a large window at standing eye level for the staff to oversee patients inside the room, a special 180-degree pivoting hinge and a double-sized door frame with a lock system either side. This system allowed the door to be secured key-locked by staff in a fixed position, either close or open, according to daily routines (to avoid patients staying/not staying in their room at certain times), and for security reasons (the door was secured to avoid accidentally or purposely hitting against anyone who could be in the corridor). Photo by Francesca Lanz, April 2022.

Asylums had been unique buildings also in way they influenced life within and beyond their walls. They were introverted spaces that separated, classified and organised people, determining patterns of life, movements, living habits and behaviours for those who lived and worked there. Asylums were 'total institutions', as Enrich Goffman defined them, i.e. institutions 'that are encompassing to a degree discontinuously greater than the ones next in line. Their encompassing or total character is symbolized by the barrier to social intercourse with the outside and to departure that is often built right into the physical plant, such as locked doors, high walls, barbed wire, cliffs, water, forest or moors' (Goffman 1961 (2007): 4). Recent studies and historical research, however, also demonstrated that they were also far more permeable than previously imagined, and deeply and variously tangled in the social and economic life of their proximate communities, not least for their remarkable size (Coleborne 2020; Coleborne and MacKinnon 2003; Gibbeson 2020; Moon et al. 2015; Topp et al. 2007).

During the 19th and 20th centuries, asylums' architectural complexes developed and spread across Europe, growing in number and, crucially, in size and influenced the architectural and urban growth of the surrounding areas, as well as their social and economic development. Those located within a city's walls were often as large as, and sometimes larger than, many of the city's major public buildings, such as the cathedral or the city hall. Those on the outskirts grew even bigger thanks to the availability of land. Asylums' influences on local development were not only due to their size, but also to the fact they were major public infrastructures, providing a wide variety of services to the local population, as well as an important source of revenue and employment. Asylums, remarks Catherine Coleborne, 'were immersed in worlds of the wider communities; they were significant in the lives of large number of people for almost the whole of the twentieth century' (2020: 3). For years, they constituted the only public option in support of individuals and their relatives struggling with mental health issues, offering subsistence, care and even forms of a sort of education to individuals. In time, they became part of the social and cultural life of their proximate communities, their identity and that of the place where they were, and soon also started developing an identity their own. They became part of local slang and ways of saying of the stories of places as well as of tall tales circulating within the local communities. Asylums have had core functions within their social, ethical and political contexts by providing touchstones for collectivities to form shared references for their identities, and encapsulating feelings of togetherness in their proximate communities. From such a perspective, their closure was in many regards a 'rupture', in Coleborne's words, for it was a dramatic and significant change for communities and individuals, and a loss of community purpose and identity (Kearns et al. 2012).

The rise and fall of the asylum

As asylums spread across Europe and beyond and kept growing rapidly in both number and scale, so did the number of their inmates. The growth of the San Lazzaro asylum in the municipality of Reggio Emilia (Italy) from its establishment in the early 19th century to the mid-20th century is representative of asylums' expansion. Already comprising 20 buildings at the beginning of the 20th century, the San Lazzaro expanded to incorporate over 40 buildings and, in the process, it became a sort of self-sufficient town on the outskirts of the small city. Within 30 years of its opening, the number of patients at the San Lazzaro had increased a hundred-fold, growing from 21 in 1825 to 233 in 1855. A large share of these were chronic patients with no hope of remission and dismissal. The population kept growing in the following decades: 599 patients in 1877, 932 in 1900, 1,428 in 1921, 1,848 in 1925, 2,123 in 1938 and eventually reaching 2,150 in 1959.[5] Similar patterns in admission and architectural expansion were common to all asylums across Europe. Initially a reflection of the great trust invested in these institutions, the growth of asylums however soon went out of control, eventually becoming one, if not the main, cause of their decline and final closure.

In the same period, the asylum population grew not only in number but also in its social and medical heterogeneity, comprising patients of different age, sex and provenance suffering from different forms of mental health issues, and with different needs and recovery prospects: from children to the elderly, including people suffering from dementia, post-traumatic stress disorders, post-partum depression, general paresis caused by syphilis, Down's syndrome, hysteria, melancholia, severe forms of schizophrenia, compulsive and paranoid disorders and much more. At the San Lazzaro asylum, for example, 5,704 former soldiers suffering from mental health problems were admitted during and immediately after WWI. Among the patients admitted in the same period were also people of various races, origins and social ranks, originating in different parts of Italy and from beyond the border, including patients displaced from other hospitals due to war and several patients suffering from post-traumatic stress following the trauma of war experiences and forced migrations.[6] Some of them, with time and care, remitted and could be dismissed, but many did not, relentlessly swelling the numbers of chronic and incurable patients and steadily increasing the average length of stay of those hospitalised in asylums. 'It was this horde of the hopeless, and the associated spectre of chronicity – notes Andrew Scull – that came to haunt late 19th century psychiatry, and to influence the larger view of the nature of madness' (2011: 55).

As might be expected, the growth in the number and heterogeneity of people admitted to asylums and their concomitant growth in size and complexity meant that running costs also increased. But staff numbers and their training did not, nor did the investment into the asylums' structures and activities. As a consequence, the quality of care and treatment provided by asylums declined drastically in a very short time, initiating a downward spiral that proved difficult to reverse. Overcrowded with people of different kinds and with little hope for remittal, and systematically understaffed and underfunded, doctors and staff increasingly struggled to provide appropriate care. The faith in the curative ability of the asylum started to waver among the wider public and also within medical sphere, while psychiatry was gradually abandoning its 19th-century optimism (Babini 2011; Porter 2002; Scull 2011).

Toward the end of the 19th century, theories about the biological origin and genetic roots of mental illness had started to find their way within the medical debate.[7] At the same time, in Germany, medical science started forming a strong bond with universities and laboratories, developing research that produced remarkable advancements in the field of brain pathologies. Among these studies were those by Alois Alzheimer (1856–1926) and Emil Kraepelin (1856–1926) that made a great contribution to modern psychiatry and became part of clinical orthodoxy. However, in practice, such progress had very little impact on the care and cure of those who were living in the asylum, who were mainly seen as a source of clinical case studies. Ironically, such studies and their findings even ended up reinforcing pessimistic views on the possibility of a cure for mental illness, paving the way to eugenic theories – of which, incidentally, Kraepelin himself was a supporter. At the outset of the 20th century, the promises and expectations placed on the reformed asylum were already vanishing. To many, the psychiatrist seemed to have been 'reduced to acting as society's policeman or gatekeeper, protecting it from the insane' (Porter 2002: 186); the role of psychiatric institutions increasingly shifted from care to social control, custody and surveillance and the rationale for their continuation mostly remained that of confinement. Meanwhile ideas on the heritable nature of madness, diffused rapidly beyond the medical sphere into politics and public opinion, supported by Social Darwinist ideas and echoed by literature and fiction, which helped them in reaching out to the wider public, contributing to the formation of many harmful stereotyped ideas and imaginaries regarding mental illness that are still, today, hard to dismantle (Mandelli 2019; Rondinone 2019).

It was not long before radical measures were suggested and actually implemented as solutions to eradicate madness from society. These included isolation in asylums with a veto on marriage for psychiatric patients, up to compulsory forced sterilisation of those deemed as insane. Andrew Scull reports that in 1940, 40 of the 48 U.S. states provided by law for compulsory sterilisation for the mentally ill (Scull 2011: 58–65). In Europe, from 1933, the Nazi regime implemented involuntary sterilisation, castration and marriage control amongst those German citizens classified as genetically defective, in the name of racial hygiene. This included people diagnosed with schizophrenia, depression disorders, epileptics, alcoholics and those born blind and deaf. Mass-murdering was to be the next step. In 1939, Adolf Hitler ratified the *Aktion T4,* also known as the *Euthanasia Programme,* which called for the 'mercy killing' of those whose life was 'not worth to be lived'.[8]

Although in Italy under the fascist regime, a similar programme was never actually implemented; during those years, the asylum became a political instrument and a tool for social and political cleansing just the same. It has been calculated that during the fascist regime almost 300 German citizens hospitalised in Italian asylums were deported to German concentration camps and thousands of people – about 30,000 – died in asylums due to lack of care. The asylums became a dark hole where the state could conveniently hide anyone who was considered troublesome or 'deviant', including also political opponents, with the silent (when not active) complicity of superintendent doctors and main psychiatric medical boards and national associations (Babini 2011).

The early 20th century, however, was also a period of key medical discoveries in central and continental Europe, that would radically change the face of asylums and mental health hospitals in the wake of the Second World War. Within the new microbiological studies, effects of bacterial infection on brain and treatment to counterstrike them were identified for the first time, including a cure for syphilis (1910) and a treatment for the general paresis of the insane (GPI) (1917) by Julius von Wagner-Jauregg (1857–1940). This meant that patients diagnosed with GPI could now be treated and cured in settings other than asylums. In those same years, other therapies based on externally provoked physiological shock were also experimented with, as possible therapies against several mental illness diagnoses. The use of barbiturates was introduced in the 1920s; insulin shock therapies and insulin-induced comas against schizophrenia were introduced in the 1930s; and electro convulsive therapy (ECT) was invented in 1938 by the Italian neuropsychiatrist Ugo Cerletti (1877–1963). Psychosurgery started developing, too. Following advances in neurophysiology and surgery practices, interventions of 'surgical bacteriology' were experimented with, including the removal of teeth, tonsils and internal organs, and lobotomy. Leucotomy techniques[9] initially won a positive appraisal among many asylums' doctors, as a possible and a viable way to 'turn no-hope asylums into true hospitals [...] and thus provide a lifeline for the [psychiatric] discipline back into mainstream general medicine' (Porter 2002: 204). Most of these treatments proved to be extremely wrong and to be great medical mistakes. Although some historians, such as Porter, point out how these medical attempts could be seen as a proof of the 'wish of well-meaning psychiatrists' who were acting at the best of their intention and within the limitation of the science of the time 'to do something for psychiatrics' forgotten patients' (*ibid.*), it is undeniable that they were grotesque and brutal. Not only were they often ineffective, but, in many cases, they worsened patients' conditions up to causing their death. What is worse is that these highly invasive treatments were experimented and administered on unwilling, vulnerable and undefended patients with little, or no, professional opposition.

In the second half of the 20th century, neuroleptics and antipsychotic drugs were to change the asylum forever. Following experiments with the use of amphetamines in the 1930s, the first psychotropic drug was introduced in 1949 for manic depression, to be followed by antipsychotic and antidepressant drugs in the 1950s and by tranquilizers in the 1970s. Chlorpromazine, which affects manic and psychotic states, was discovered in 1951 by the French neurosurgeon Henri Laborit (1914–1995) and it was commercialised as *Largactil* and *Thorazine* two years later, bringing an astonishing transformation to Paris asylums, where 'violence, shouting, disruptive behaviours and straitjacket had all melted way, replaced by calm, silence and daily injections' (Jay 2016: 176). The new drugs did not cure mental illness, but they made it manageable. The advent of the use of neuroleptics and antipsychotic drugs provided much-needed support for mental hospital nurses and staff and made it possible to refocus on patients' wellbeing. Since then, it has become evident that drugs were a far from perfect solution. It can prove very difficult to find the proper dosage and, even so, they can cause disrupting side effects including dizziness, indolence, uncontrolled weight gain, muscle stiffening and dependency up to emotional flattening and the patient's dehumanisation. The use of drugs inadvertently created space for other types of abuses on patients, who were once again restrained and silenced, this time chemically, and forced to undergo therapies against their will – medicated rather than cared for (Barham 2020). However, when they were first introduced, these drugs helped to drastically reduce the number of people being institutionalised. Instead, these people could be sent home or treated in other settings, possibly better – and mistakenly thought as less expensive – than previous ones. It became possible to envision a future without asylums.

Open criticism of the asylum started to emerge in the 1950s coming from both thinkers and psychiatrists themselves, with the work of Foucault and Goffman being seminal reference points (Foucault 1961; Goffman 1961). These critics were soon to be followed by more and more radical ones addressed not only against the asylum but towards psychiatry itself (Crossley 1998; 2006). Nick Crossley defines them as 'revolts' (Crossley 1998). The 'revolt from without', constituted by the non-specialistic attacks on psychiatry, mainly those made by the Church of Scientology between the 1950s and 1980s; the 'revolt from below', represented by the birth and growth of the user/survivor movement in the United Kingdom in the 1970s; and the most crucial one, at least in its implications for the future of the asylum, the 'revolt from above' of the 'anti-psychiatric' movement, which emerged in the 1960s and 1970s. 'Antipsychiatry' is a term first used by the psychiatrist and theorist David Cooper (1931–1986) in 1967. His ideas were taken up and further developed in the following decades in Europe and United States within the international socio-cultural context of counterculture and under the influence of the work of several charismatic thinkers and psychiatrists, such as David Cooper himself and Ronald David Laing in the United Kingdom, Thomas Szasz in Hungary and Franco Basaglia in Italy – although some of them, including Laing and Basaglia, would later reject the term 'antipsychiatry'. As Crossley articulates, 'anti-psychiatrists, in contrast to previous and many subsequent critics, did not question particular treatments or policies, nor did they simply argue for a more humane psychiatry [...] they questioned the very basis of psychiatry itself: its purpose, its foundational conception of mental illness and the very distinction between madness and sanity itself' (*Ibid.*, 878).

Meanwhile, the way the general population looked at and thought about the asylum had started to change. At their inception, the internment in these structures was intended to be curative, based on medical treatments, informed by reason, science and moral therapies and its aim was patients' cure, rehabilitation and their return into society. Their loss of freedom, as Susanne Piddock highlights, was meant to be, in principle, temporary, due to a momentary loss of reason, and therefore it was considered 'acceptable and justified', for it was 'in the best interest of the individual concerned' (Piddock 2007: 11). Those who could afford otherwise, had always tried to avoid the asylum. Whenever possible, the well-to-do usually preferred other sorts of arrangements for relatives in need of mental care, such as a foreign retreat, if for no other reason than to escape the shame and the 'gossiping' that came with asylum hospitalisation. By the early 20th century, however, the asylum was starting to be regarded with increasing scepticism and even anxiety within the public opinion at large. On top of the actual decline of the quality of care provided within many of these institutions, contributing factors for this scepticism were asylum isolation and the lack of knowledge about life within its walls, the increasingly extended lengths of internments and the many hindrances to visiting loved ones who were hospitalised, which nurtured dark speculations and gruesome imaginaries about what could happen in the asylum.

In 1970–1971, hundreds of people organised several non-authorised incursions at the San Lazzaro asylum in Reggio Emilia to check on the status and condition of their family members, fellow countrymen and women who were detained there (Babini 2011; Foot 2014: 228–232). Known as '*le calate*', such initiatives were supported and backed up by radical psychiatrists, trade unionists, activists and local left-wing party members. The first one took place in 1970 and involved a group of about 40 citizens from Ramiseto a small village located on the mountain area surrounding the city of Reggio Emilia. On the 23rd of November 1970, they rented a bus and 'went down' to town to visit the asylum: they caught the superintendent doctor and the staff by surprise and once inside the asylum they were confronted with a grim situation, which was particularly shocking in the child ward with little children fastened in beds and highchairs. Pictures taken during the burst-in were circulated in the public domain and a huge scandal followed. It is still debated whether and how the *calate* actually contributed to improving the situation within the San Lazzaro asylum. However, they were clearly emblematic of an ongoing, radical change in the way asylums were regarded by the public as well in the medical and in the political sphere.

In those same years, the cost-cutting imperative and the radical reassessment of welfare and mental healthcare systems of late 20th century meant that the asylum was increasingly considered as an unsuitable and unsustainable option for ministering to the mentally ill. Undermined in both medical and political opinion, overcome in their approaches and scope by new medical advancements, overcrowded, ill-run, over-expensive and under-funded, the era of the asylum was coming to an end.

The turn of the 1960s saw the height of 'deinstitutionalisation'. This term indicates a post–Second World War trend across Europe and overseas, gradually emptying out, running-down and closing traditional mental hospitals and, instead, seeking the least restrictive treatments possible, with community care seen as an alternative to prolonged hospitalisation (Barham 2020; Paulson 2012). Although enthusiastically supported by politicians seeking a way to shrink the asylum, streamline its services and reduce costs, deinstitutionalisation was first and foremost a revolution driven by the genuine desire to improve and advance treatments and provision offered to people struggling with mental health. It aimed for a new and more effective model and approach to the management of and ministering to those considered insane, that could offer a viable alternative to the asylum as the primary mode of care. The search for a *significantly better* model was equated with the implementation of a *substantially different* one. The asylum was rejected for its authoritarian, subjugating and potentially abusive nature, based on an understanding of mental illness as deviance, and it was believed that a viable and better alternative might lie in the new drugs and in a community-based caring system, equally hinged on public welfare provision and social accountability.

Whilst deinstitutionalisation was an international phenomenon accompanied by a lively international scholarly and scientific debate, there has never been a single, coherent cross-national policy of deinstitutionalisation. The closure of the asylums, happened in different ways in different countries and it was indeed a fraught and uneven process, that followed very different trajectories and that led to very different outcomes across European countries and overseas. Nowadays, in most European countries, many mental asylums have evolved into psychiatric hospitals that are still up and running, although considerably downscaled, restructured in their way of working and flanked by other forms of provision (mainly community-based approaches, such as therapeutic communities and assisted residential units). Despite sometimes remarkable differences in each country's specific regulations, involuntary admission to a mental health facility and compulsory administering of treatments is still possible in several countries across Europe.[10] Italy is a unique exception; there, all psychiatric hospitals of any kind, including forensic ones, have been closed by law, following the ratification of the law, no. 180 in 1978, commonly known as the *Legge Basaglia* (Babini 2011; Foot 2014).[11]

The complete closure of mental hospitals in Italy took years to be implemented and in most cases patients remained in the asylum waiting for a long time for a better location, with the last patients dismissed only in the late 1990s. Similarly, in other countries that opted for a less radical approach than the Italian one, deinstitutionalisation was a gradual process rather than a sudden shift. Nevertheless, it was in many regards a 'rupture' – as Catherine Colborne calls it – inasmuch it was in effect a deep and wholesale break with the past and in some case event violent and traumatic (2020). Indeed, while for many the closure of the asylums was a timely, necessary and inevitable step forward towards a more humane and progressive approach to the care of mental illness; still, for others, it was a challenge and a loss. Some members of the medical staff were reluctant to accept a change that was seen as not only redefining their consolidated ways of working and practices, sometimes drastically, but also somehow questioning their role, skills and professionalism. This created resistance and tensions among those working in the mental health sectors within asylums. There was also resistance to change among asylums' proximate communities. This was due to preoccupations for the possible disruptions caused by the closure of such large public infrastructures, the potential drop in services and jobs and the release of former asylums' patients into neighbouring communities, which in some cases was regarded as a possible threat to social security. Resistance came also from the perceived loss of 'purpose and identity' across such communities which for many years had been, in effect, bound to the local asylum, not least because often a large share of the local population had been working for and at the asylum for years, sometimes for several generations, developing sometimes rewarding careers and forming friendships and personal relations with patients and other staff members (Gibbeson 2020; Kearns et al. 2012). Opposition was raised, although only lately, by policy makers and policy advisors, who, after a more accurate assessment of its financial implications, started to realise how the shift to community-based model did not in reality reconcile with the political and economic policies of cost containment that were amongst its grounding rationales. Resistance and reservations could be found among asylum patients and their families, too. For some, their dismissal from hospital to community care was a liberation from a demeaning place of suffering and abuse, and the restitution of freedom and dignity; for others it was, in effect, the loss of a secure place to live in the absence of any other lodging, means of subsistence and aid. Equally, for some families, closure of asylums offered the possibility of reunion with loved ones, but for others, it meant taking over a psychological and practical burden of ministering to severely mentally unstable relatives with little, if any, support.

Thus, the process of deinstitutionalisation was anything but unanimous. The fierce criticism of the asylum could be thus seen as being aimed at 'vilifying' the asylum (Moon et al. 2015) to undermine possible opposition to its closure through a sometimes exaggerated and 'denigratory campaign' (Franklin 2002a) that drew upon asylums' actual states of deterioration, further worsened by journalists, sociologists, Hollywood filmmakers and even many of the psychiatric profession. The very length of the implementation of the deinstitutionalisation process might be linked back not only to its practical difficulties, but also as deliberately and conveniently prolonged in time to mollify possible oppositions. As Moon, Kearns and Alun articulate, 'the protracted nature of the "real" as opposed to the "formal" processes of closing psychiatric asylums served in most instances to dilute and deflect public debate (as well as media interest) in the demise of these previously-prominent institutions' (Moon et al. 2015: 17). Although it took years, following the deinstitutionalisation process and the 'psychiatric revolutions' of the mid-20th century, the change from asylums to a combination of care in the community and psychiatric hospitals also led to a reconsideration of the psychiatric services that institutions should provide. Broadly speaking, the variety of types of services offered has been considerably downscaled, mostly limited to providing assistance and beds for those suffering from acute and severe cases of mental illness. Among other things, this meant that former 19th-century asylums' large architectural complexes had become increasingly medically, socially, functionally and architecturally obsolete, and therefore they had been progressively disused.

Palimpsests[12]

Volterra is a small town in Tuscany, Italy. Today, it is an internationally renowned tourist destination for its fine food and wine and its Etruscan and mediaeval heritage; however, it was once famous for its alabaster quarries and it's mad'. Once, in fact, Volterra hosted one of the biggest and most peculiar asylums in Italy: the San Girolamo asylum.

Established in the early 19th century, 1 kilometre south of the town's walls; even before the Second World War, the San Girolamo had a capacity of over 4,000 patients within an estate comprising 25 buildings, as well as extensive farmland and fields extending more than 300 hectares (Ajroldi et al. 2013: 207–208; *Gli Spazi della Follia*, n.d. [Last Accessed, September 2022]). Because of its remarkable size – which becomes even more remarkable when compared to the relatively small dimensions of Volterra – the asylum was one of the major employers in the area and an economic cornerstone for the small town, as essential to the local economy as the alabaster quarries. Crucially, in time, it also became an important element of the life and identity of the city and its local population.

What distinguished the San Girolamo asylum was not only its dimensions, but also its unique approach to the care and management of its inmates. The San Girolamo asylum was once one of the most pioneering and progressive asylums in Italy, possibly across Europe, for its genuinely experimental community-based therapeutic approach and radical no-restraint policy. This was introduced during the first decades of the 20th century under the direction of the superintendent doctor Luigi Scabia,[13] and continued to be developed into the 1980s, during the post-deinstitutionalisation period. Mainly informed by Scabia's vision, the asylum was conceived and run as a village – self-sufficient but open and strongly interwoven with Volterra's socio-economic life and identity. Quite unusually, in Volterra, there was no physical separation, containment wall or fence enclosing and isolating the asylum from the city; rather, there were continuous and two-way exchanges between them. Several patients, for example, were allowed out of the asylum perimeter during the daytime. It was usual to meet them walking down the town's streets or sitting on the benches and stop for a quick chat with them; some patients contributed to the city's maintenance as part of their occupational therapy. Most of them were known by name; on special occasions, local families sometimes hosted patients or their family members, and some of them eventually created lasting friendships. Emblematically, for a time, the asylum even issued its own coins, which could be spent by the patients in local shops and then paid back either in cash or in kind by the asylum admin.

In Volterra, the proximity of the asylum and its patients was not merely tolerated; in their own way, they were integrated among the local population. Because a large share of the relatively small local population worked at the hospital, the asylum had a core function within Volterra's social, ethical and political context by providing a touchstone for the local community to form shared references for identities, encapsulating and fostering feelings of togetherness that further reinforced the already quite strong local sense of community and belonging. Volterra asylum's 'open' model and the fact that several doctors, nurses and staff members honestly sought, within the limits of their capacity, alternative and more humane models of care for the asylum's inmates, remains today a source of pride among the local former asylum staff community and their relatives.

Despite the pioneering and progressive approach that characterised psychiatric practices implemented there, San Girolamo was far from a perfect 'fairy-tale' place. The relentless increase in the number of patients admitted to the asylum was not matched by an adequate increase in funding, staff training and medical equipment. This resulted in an inexorable decrease in the quality of care and treatment provided. As with many other asylums across the country and abroad, systematic overcrowding and underfinancing paved the way for negligence, misconduct and abuses, resulting in incredibly harsh and often inhumane living conditions for patients and extremely challenging working conditions for staff members. Following the ratification of the *Legge Basaglia*, the San Girolamo asylum started to be gradually shut down. Meanwhile, alternative forms of therapy and community-based care were explored and implemented; patients were slowly either discharged or relocated into other structures. Staff who could not be made redundant by contract were reassigned to other duties at different facilities in the area, and the asylum buildings were gradually emptied out and disused. Today, the asylum is closed. Some pavilions have been demolished; others were converted for the public health system. A few pavilions were sold for residential development, but this was never realised and, today, like most of the other buildings of the complex, they are just abandoned and in an advanced state of decay.

Part of the asylum estate today can be visited with a guided tour, which I attended during my fieldwork, together with a group of research participants.[14] The tour started as part of a Urbex project promoted by the UE association, *I Luoghi dell'Abbandono* [The Places of Abandonment].[15] Today, the guided walk is part of the activities promoted by the local cultural association, *Inclusione Graffio e Parola*[16] [Inclusion Scratch and Word], which is also in charge of running and managing a small asylum museum, named *Museo Lombroso,* and hosted in one of the former asylum pavilions named after Cesare Lombroso. *Inclusione Graffio e Parola* is a not-for-profit organisation founded in 2010 by a group of volunteers, including several former nurses and their family members, with the chief objective to preserve and valorise the asylum's heritage and in particular the graffiti by a patient, Oreste Fernando Nannetti alias NOF4 (Miorandi 2022), realised on the interior and exterior walls of the two San Girolamo asylum's forensic pavilions, the Ferri and the Charcot. Nannetti's work is today recognised as a major example of 'art brute'.[17] The asylum is very near the city centre but there are practically no signposts pointing tourists to its location and the tour is mostly promoted via word of mouth and social media. The visit mainly consists of a walk in the former asylum complex, which material remnants, notably including NOF4's graffiti, are used by the guide as the support and starting point to recount the asylum's history and the life in there. We walked in the asylum estate, which once housed the asylum gardens, decorated with trees, flower beds and fountains, and today is reclaimed by wild, untamed nature. We passed by several former pavilions, once obviously magnificent, now crumbling and dilapidated, their walls covered with murals and writings and inaccessible because of their extremely precarious and dangerous condition. What was once a site of noise (MacKinnon 2011) is today pervaded by an alien silence, the twittering of cicadas and the squeaking and creaking of the old pavilions falling apart. The atmosphere is extremely emotive. It is no surprise that the asylum has become popular among Urban Explorers and extensively featured on several Urbex websites, such as *I luoghi dell'abbandono* and *Ascosi Lasciti*.[18] The place atmosphere and history has also nurtured rich cultural and artistic responses, such as Marina Abramovic's site-specific performance *Mambo a Marienbad* [Mambo in Marienbad], designed for and performed in the Charcot pavilion, or 1984 Paolo Rosa's film *L'osservatorio nucleare del sig.Nanof* [The Nuclear Observatory of Mr Nanof] shot in the asylum premises.

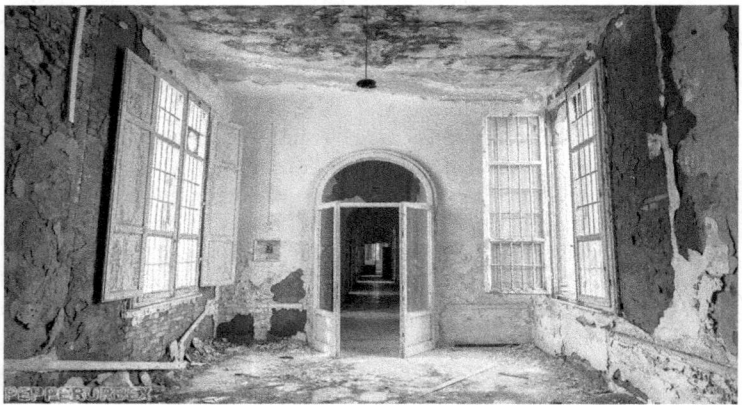

Image 1.4 The San Girolamo asylum in Volterra in a photo by the Dutch urban explorer 'Pepper', November 18th, 2018.
We read in the text accompanying the images: 'Looking like something straight out of a horror movie, the Ospedale Psichiatrico di Volterra is the crumbling husk of a mental institution that was closed due to cruel treatment of its patients, one of whom left a mysterious work of epic scale etched into the plaster of the walls that imprisoned him'. Source: https://pepperurbex.com/ [Last Accessed, October 2022]. Photo courtesy of Theo Zwart.

During the visit, one could easily imagine the beauty of the site and its buildings as they were once back in time. The architecture of the asylum, its pavilions and outdoor spaces, harks back to the 19th-century idea of the asylum as a curative, therapeutic and healing place. The apex of the visit is at the Ferri pavilion, where NOF4's graffiti are. The architectural style of the Ferri pavilion is similar to the one of the other asylum buildings: a two-storey pavilion with double-arched windows. Unlike the other pavilions and in contrast with the overall design of the asylum, the Ferri pavilion features bars at its windows, individual cells with security doors and the remains of the double fence wall with barbed wire fence that once surrounded it. In the yard, still there are tables and benches made of solid concrete and firmly fixed to the ground, arranged in the space to impede any modification and allow the nurses and guards to have complete visual control over the patients and the activities taking place there.

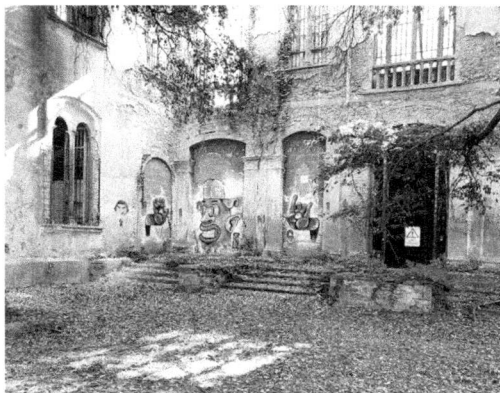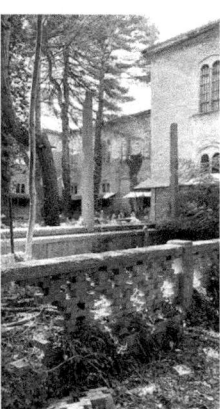

Image 1.5 The Ferri pavilion, photo by Eleonora Anna Scigliano (research participant, August 2021).
The Ferri pavilion was built in 1934 as the asylum forensic pavilion, following the ratification of the 1904 *Legge Giolitti*. The number of inmates in the Ferri grew from 350 in 1934 to over 1,000 in only five years, with a nurse-patient ratio of 1 to 30. Among patients interned at the Ferri, there was Fernando Oreste Nannetti, author of the graffiti that covers a large part of the pavilion interior and exterior walls. It features remnants of its former double containment wall and iron barbed fence, demolished in 1972. The pavilion is today inaccessible due to its precarious conditions and it has suffered from structural collapses and human-caused damages. Photo courtesy of Eleonora Anna Scigliano.

The Ferri was the asylum forensic ward and was built from 1930–1933 in compliance with the 1904 *Legge Giolitti*. NOF4's graffiti unfolds on the Ferri exterior wall, going round windows, wall decorations and

wall-mounted fixed furniture. Sometimes they take the shape of silhou-
ettes; these are the outlines of some of his fellow patients, who were so
alienated that they sat every day on the same bench, practically
motionless. Nannetti carved his daily diary around them, as if they were
part of the architecture of the place. After the pavilion closure, it has been
abandoned and left to decay; under the effect of neglect, weathering and
deliberate abuse and vandalism, the pavilion and the graffiti deteriorated
fast and, in recent years, many among the local population started to take
action in order to raise awareness amongst the local authorities of the
site's historical relevance and to promote its preservation and valorisation,
as the activities of the association *Inclusione Graffio e Parola* and the
project *Manicomio di Volterra* [The Asylum of Volterra].[19]

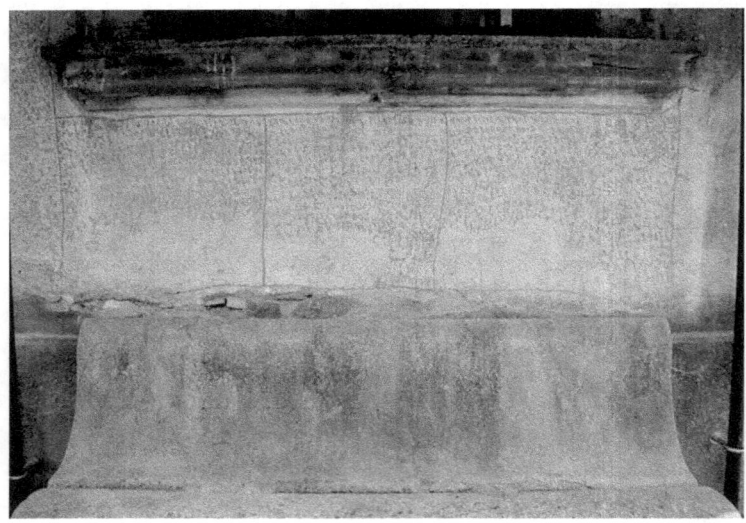

Image 1.6 NOF4 graffiti at the Ferri pavilion, photo by Gloria Marchetti, 2012.
The graffiti in the pavilion's yard originally covered a surface 180 m long and
about 2 m high, extending over the exterior walls of the pavilion, where Nannetti
was detained from 1958 to 1973. It consists of a bustrofedic text[20] composed of
images and words carved every day on the plaster of the wall by Nannetti during
his time out using his uniform's waistcoat buckle to annotate anything he
considered worthy in his diary of the asylum life. Photo courtesy of Gloria
Marchetti.

During my visit to Volterra, I met Alice Ceppatelli and Alessandro
Massi for the first time. Alice was born and raised in Volterra; it has been
her family's home for generations. During our time together, Alice and
Alessandro recounted to me anecdotes and episodes of daily life in

Volterra that gave a vivid sense of how much the asylum was a part of the town, for good and bad. Alice herself has a strong personal and emotional attachment to the site, and to NOF4's graffiti in particular. She told me about her granddad, who was a nurse at the hospital and used to walk his dogs in the asylum estate after the end of his shift to 'check on it'. She told me about her and her friends' nighttime incursions into the abandoned site as a test of courage, and about the time she went down to Rome to retrace the places of Nannetti's life. She showed me her tattoos inspired by NOF4's artworks. Alice feels the asylum to be a key part of her identity as a 'Volterrana'. Alessandro has also developed a strong sense of attachment to the San Girolamo; to him, it encapsulates the open and inclusive spirit of Volterra, from which he does not originate but where he feels he belongs 'by adoption'. Alice and Alessandro have turned their interest and passion for the site into a project called *Manicomio di Volterra*. They research and collect memories and stories of the asylum and share them through their website and associated social platforms, including a Facebook group with almost 3,000 members.[21] The aim of the project is to 'collect, promote and communicate information, memories and stories about the former asylum' and 'prevent the loss of the memory of this place at risk of neglect' (*Manicomio di Volterra* website, Last Accessed, October 2022).

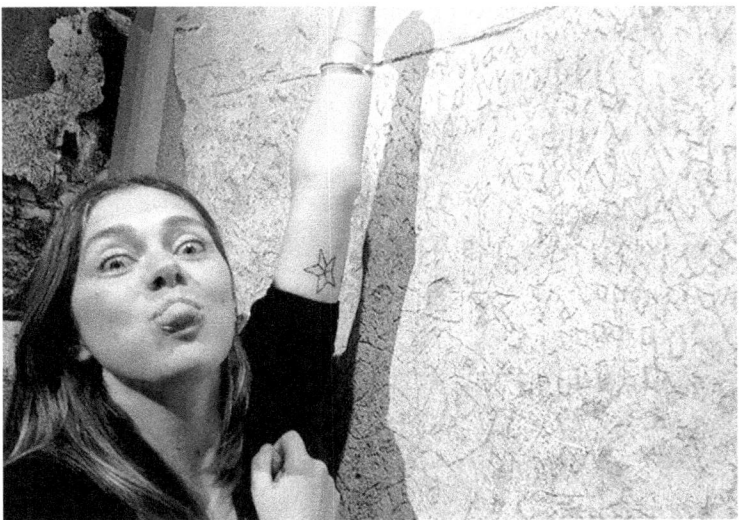

Image 1.7 Alice Ceppatelli.
Shoot taken at the *Museo Lombroso*, in Volterra, in the room where NOF4's graffiti are on display. Photo by Alessandro Massi; courtesy of Alessandro Massi and Alice Ceppatelli.

The San Girolamo case exemplifies how, since its inception throughout its life span and over the years, several memories, meanings and agendas might converge and coalesce on an architectural assemblage, erasing, rewriting, overlapping, sometimes competing and conflicting with one another. It is quite evident how at the Volterra asylum all and each of these actions have made a palimpsest of this site. It is a cumulative and meaning palimpsest, as per Bailey's definition (2007), or, we may say a palimpsest of 'traces', understood by Jon Anderson's interpretation, as 'marks, residues or remnants, left in place by cultural life' (Anderson 2021: 8). Traces – says Anderson – can equally be smaller or larger physical leftovers, as well as memories, events, or emotions. Whatever their nature, however, traces last and endure in time: they can be seen, sensed or thought about. Furthermore, he remarks, traces 'are constantly produced'; 'they continually influence the meaning and identity of places'. In that, 'they function as connections, tying the meaning of places to the identity of the cultural groups who make them' (*ibid.*, 9). At the San Girolamo as in many other similar former asylum sites, these traces in their accumulation tie the past to the present in a continuous process of making and becoming, which discloses its yet unfulfilled potential as places of awareness.

Notes

1 See note no. 4 in the Introduction.
2 For a critical discussion on the cultural and political role of Pinel and Tuke in the birth of the asylum and the myth of the "liberation of the insane" and the differences between their 'moral approaches', respectively, ration- and religion-based see Foucault's chapter on the 'Birth of the Asylum' (1961 (2006): 465–511).
3 They notably include Philippe Pinel himself; the English Quakers William Tuke (1732–1822) and his grandson Samuel Tuke (1784–1857), who founded the York Retreat, one of the first and most pioneering examples of a facility for the care and treatment of people with mental health issues, conceived and run following a religious-based moral approach (Tuke 1813); Vittorio Chiarugi (1759–1820) in Florence, who was the first alienist substituting chains with soft restraints and pioneer of the psychiatric reform in a not-yet-unified Italy under the auspices of the Gran Duke Pietro Leopoldo; and Johan Christian Reil (1759–1813) in Germany, who first coined the term 'psychiatry'.
4 An early example is the Narrenturm in Vienna, a purposely built tower, 5 storeys high with 139 cells disposed in a radial layout realised in Vienna 1784 to host mad people and disused in the late 1790s with the rise of the moral reform approach. Today, the Narrenturm is one of the venues of *Wien Natural History Museum*, hosting and displaying a collection of anatomical pathology and offering guided tours covering the history of the site.
   Another rare example of panopticon pavilion in a 19th-century asylum complex is the Conolly pavilion at the San Niccolò asylum in Siena in Tuscany, Italy (Angrisano 2019; Colucci 2007). The pavilion was designed by the architect Francesco Azzurri and inaugurated in 1876. The pavilion is the only remaining example of a panopticon pavilion with a medical purpose in Italy and one of the few worldwide; today, it lies in a state of abandonment and advanced decay.

5 Architectural data from the online portals *Gli Spazi della Follia* [Last Accessed, August 2022]; data on admission and patients from the online database *Carte da Legare* (Direzione Generale Archivi n.d. [Last Accessed, August 2022]).

6 Data on admission and patients from the online database *Carte da Legare* (Direzione Generale Archivi n.d. [Last Accessed, August 2022]). The Law no. 36, dated 14th February 1904 (the so-called *Legge Giolitti* that regulated Italian asylum admission until the *Legge Basaglia* was ratified in 1978) read: 'Everyone who for whatever reason is affected by any form of mental derangement shall be kept in a mental asylum, whenever they are dangerous for themselves or others, or they are a cause of public scandal, and they are not and cannot be watched and cured in other settings than an asylum'.

7 Already in the mid-19th century, the French alienist Bénédict Morel (1809–1873) introduced the concept of 'degeneration.' In those same years, the Italian psychiatrist Cesare Lombroso (1835–1909) developed theories on the biological origin of criminal behaviours, forging a branch of science that was to be termed 'anthropological criminology'. Anthropological criminology was based on physiognomy and phrenology, atavistic degenerationism and Darwinism, and revolved around the assumption of a direct and detectable relationship between criminal psychopathology and physical or constitutional defects. According to Lombroso's theory, not only was it possible to identify people's natural inclinations to deviance through the study of their somatic traits, but this was part of their nature; some people were 'born criminal'. Lombroso's ideas proved to be wrong and his theories lacking any scientific support and credibility; he was even eventually expelled by the *Società Italiana di Antropologia ed Etnologia* – the Italian Scientific Association for Anthropology and Ethnology – in 1882. Nevertheless, his theories spread, rapidly influencing psychiatric practices and ideas on the incurability and genetic inferiority of people suffering from mental health problems. These ideas proved to be enduring and they were to be taken over into the following century within and beyond the medical sphere.

8 The expression from Nazi propaganda was 'life unworthy of life'; in German: *Lebensunwertes Leben.*

The *Aktion T4* was the first mass-killing programme implemented by Hitler's regime in the name of racial purity (Götz 2017; Proctor 1988). It is estimated that not less than 200,000 people with mental disabilities and mental illness were murdered by the Nazi regime from 1939 to 1945 in Germany, the occupied Poland and the territories of what is today the Czech Republic in gas chambers and through lethal injections. This largely happened with the support of doctors, within mental hospitals and church-run asylums, and in the shadow of the social isolation and physical seclusion offered by these places. Most of these atrocities have remained for a long time hidden and anonymised, even after the end of the war and still today killings of the *Aktion T4* are rarely publicly discussed and acknowledged in comparison with other crimes of the Nazi era. Aly Götz, a German journalist and historian, contends that this is largely due to the stigma, shame and taboo surrounding mental illness in the past and today, for the embarrassment of 'madness' goes over resistance, grief and even the will for due justice and recognition (2017).

9 Leucotomy, or lobotomy, was first developed in Lisbon by the neurologist Egas Moniz (1874–1955) and then taken up by Walter Freemand in Washington, DC (1895–1972).

10 General principles aimed at promoting the rights of mentally disabled persons in health care are set by the UN *Principles for the Protection of Persons with Mental Illness and the Improvement of Mental Health Care* adopted by General Assembly resolution 46/119 of 17 December 1991 (UN 1991).

11 The *Legge Basaglia* has been the first and, so far, most radical law reforming mental health care in Europe and beyond. Following the *Legge Basaglia* in Italy today, in no case can anyone be administered a treatment without their informed consent with the sole exception of people sent to Obligatory Sanitary Treatment (TSO). TSO is an extreme measure to be enforced by a doctor and a police officer and involves obligatory hospitalisation and treatment that cannot last for more than 7 days in a row – rarely extended to 15 in the most severe cases. In any other case, mental health treatments are solely and completely administered on a voluntary basis. The consequences of a sentence of incompetence, following a legal and medically supported hearing, encompass only the person's ability for independent administering of their possessions. Mental health care is fundamentally community-based, its practices are largely informed by social psychology and radical psychiatry ideas and approaches, as they were developed within the Italian movement *Psichiatria Democratica* under the leadership of the influential psychiatrist Franco Basaglia.

12 An extended version of this chapter has been published as 'The Building as a Palimpsest: Heritage, Memory and Adaptive Reuse Beyond Intervention' in the *Journal of Cultural Heritage Management and Sustainable Development* (Lanz 2023).

13 Luigi Scabia (1868–1934) was superintendent doctor at Volterra from 1900 to 1934.

14 Fieldwork and on-site workshop at Volterra former asylum, August 2021.

15 *I Luoghi dell'Abbandono* Facebook page: https://www.facebook.com/iluoghidellabbandono?locale=it_IT [Last Accessed, March 2023].

16 *Inclusione Graffio e Parola* website: https://www.inclusionegraffioeparola.it [Last Accessed, October 2022].

17 'Art brute', or 'outsider art', 'is a French term that translates as "raw art", invented by the French artist Jean Dubuffet to describe art such as graffiti or naïve art which is made outside the academic tradition of fine art' (Tate Website, https://www.tate.org.uk/art/art-terms/a/art-brut [Last Accessed, October 2022]).

18 *Ascosi Lasciti* website: https://ascosilasciti.com/it/ [Last Accessed, October 2022].

19 *Manicomio di Volterra* website https://manicomiodivolterra.it/ [Last Accessed, March 2023].

20 Bustrofedic writing is a form of bidirectional writing in which each line begins on the side where the previous one ended.

21 *Manicomio di Volterra* Facebook page https://manicomiodivolterra.it/ [Last Accessed, October 2022]. *Manicomio di Volterra* facebook group https://www.facebook.com/groups/gruppodelmanicomiodivolterra [Last Accessed, March 2023].

2 Mind museums

Asylums have left behind residues and remnants, creating complex palimpsests of traces that today coalesce, and sometimes conflict, in the contemporary landscape of the heritage of mental health. This chapter focuses on this heritage, bringing museums into sharp focus. Although it was extremely rare to find a public museum in a working asylum, forms of public display and collecting were common in these institutions since their inception. In several public madhouses, mad hospitals and asylums, it was common practice to allow in a paying public: the Bethlem asylum became notorious for that (Andrews et al. 1998: 178–199; Jay 2016: 47–56) and while public visits at Bethlem were forbidden by end of the 18th century; in other asylums, they continued for longer. During the 19th century at the San Lazzaro asylum in Reggio Emilia, for example, paying visitors were allowed in every Sunday: the superintendent doctor, Augusto Tamburini, edited a touristic guide of the asylum in 1880, which was last updated in 1900. Tourism was in fact a source of extra revenue for asylums and a means for fundraising through charity. However, even though indeed morbid curiosity, voyeurism and entertainment were reasons for visiting as much as, if not more than, duty and compassion, visiting the asylum was also meant to be a moral and educational experience, very much in light with the 18th-century Enlightenment paternalistic attitude. As Jonathan Andrews and his co-authors point out in their history of Bethlem, 'the insane were displayed as a didactic spectacle', the viewing was meant to 'impress the minds and hearts of … visitors' for it was essentially supposed to be a 'moral experience through turning the mirror' (Andrews et al. 1998: 183–184).

Precisely because of the moral implications of the spectacle of punishment involved in 18th- and 19th-century asylum visiting, as well as for the scopic regimes and the subtended power relations characterising asylum life and spaces, the asylum has been discussed in relation to museums and other institutions as part of the 'exhibitionary

DOI: 10.4324/9781003258971-3

complex' (Bennett 1998). However, as Tony Bennett himself remarks, drawing on Foucault, while asylums gradually withdrew from the public sphere to become places of incarceration, '[t]he institutions comprising "the exhibitionary complex", by contrast, were involved in the transfer of objects and bodies from the enclosed and private domains in which they had previously been displayed (but to a restricted public) into progressively more open and public arenas where, through the representations to which they were subjected, they formed vehicles for inscribing and broadcasting the messages of power (but of a different type) throughout society' (*ibid.*, 74). Asylums and museums thus constitute 'two different sets of institutions and their accompanying knowledge/power relations, then, whose histories, in these respects, run in opposing directions' (*ibid.*). The following chapter explores how the separated histories of mental asylums and museums eventually re-merged into contemporary mind museums. Here I will define in outline a mind museum by tracing its origins within 19th-century asylum collecting practices, framing their birth within the deinstitutionalisation movement, and eventually discussing their more recent development. In doing so, attention is given to exhibition design, meaning display[1] set up in a given space[2] (Dernie 2006; MacLeod et al. 2012; Tzortzi 2015; Roppola 2012). Combining a museographical approach with theories from museum studies[3] (Lanz and Leveratto 2023; Lindauer 2006; Moser 2010), the critical analysis of mind museums' exhibition design is here, intended not only to describe how mind museums are, but also to understand what they do, and thereby establishing a basis for investigating their effects – a matter that will be discussed in the concluding chapter.

Collecting, collections and the asylum

As Catherine Coleborne and Dolly MacKinnon remark in the opening chapter of their edited volume *Exhibiting Madness* – one of the few publications exploring the role of objects and material culture in the writing of histories of psychiatry – '[c]ollecting has been a driving force at the centre of the multiple functions of psychiatric institutions over their entire history' (Coleborne and Mackinnon 2011: 9). In that regard, the asylum was no different from other medical institutions of the time (Alberti 2011; Arnold 2005): if '[m]edical practitioners were among the most prolific collectors of all kinds of objects' (Alberti 2011: 20), then psychiatrists were no exception. Most asylum superintendent doctors in fact collected medical objects for both personal interest and study (Coleborne 2001; Coleborne 2003; Coleborne 2011; Coleborne 2020). In contrast to was happening in other medical institutions, however, 19th-century asylum collecting practices were not so much driven by didactic purposes as by the intent to document the evolutionary development of therapeutic practices and the medical and scientific advancements of psychiatric approaches of the time in an historical moment when psychiatry was shifting from being regarded as a shady profession to establishing itself as a recognised and authoritative medical practice and discipline. In a similar way to what Samuel Alberti remarks about medical museums and anatomy collections, collecting within the asylum can be related with what Simon Chaplin has called the 'museum œconomy' to describe 'the system of operations by which the collecting and display of preserved body parts allowed the surgeon-anatomist to represent himself as a virtuous and knowledgeable medical practitioner' (Alberti 2011: 47). At the same time, asylums collecting practices epitomised the same 'rhetoric of power' embodied in the exhibitionary complex itself: 'a power made manifest not in its ability to inflict pain but by its ability to organise and co-ordinate an order of things and to produce a place for the people in relation to that order [...] a power which aimed at a rhetorical effect through its representation of otherness rather than at any disciplinary effects' (Bennett 1998: 80).

The tradition of collecting in the asylum continued pretty much unchanged in its rationale and practices throughout the 20th century. However, while medical and anatomical collections and displays gradually evolved into medical museums by developing primarily teaching and educational purposes, this was not the case for asylums' collections. These collections never left the asylum, and they retained an essentially hybrid nature, in-between institutional and private interests, scientific collections and psychiatric cabinets of curiosity.

These collections today constitute the oldest core of mind museums' collections. The array of objects they include is extensive and heterogeneous. These typically span from medical tools, equipment and machines for different kinds of treatments, to hydrotherapy bathtubs and showers, physiotherapy chairs, syringes for insulin therapies, test tubes, lobotomy tools, X-ray machines, ophthalmoscopes, laparoscopy kits, ECT machines, straitjackets and so much more. They also usually include instruments that were already redundant by the 19th-century asylum but that had been collected as evidence of the evolution of psychiatric treatments and the medical profession compared to previous practices, most commonly chains, fetters, shackles and other tools for mechanical restraint. Furthermore, psychiatry collecting was not limited to medical objects but also involved pathological and anatomical specimens and they often included tissue slides, organs in formaldehyde and skulls, which were usually accompanied by phrenological and physiognomic studies including drawings and pathological photographic collections.

The collecting practices and collections of the 19th-century asylum also encompassed a considerable amount of heterogeneous textual resources, which were produced and accumulated by the asylum as part of its institutional and medical work. In time, they came to constitute oftentimes remarkably large archives and bibliographic collections. These archival collections typically include medical books – comprising encyclopaedias, treatises and scientific journals – and other asylum-produced texts and documents, such as superintendent doctors' diaries and reports from medical studies carried out at the asylum. Oftentimes, they also contain architectural documentation about the asylum building and its later expansions, usually asylum site plans and architectural projects, models, architectural reports and building records. In most cases, they also contain documents pertaining to the day-by-day asylum management and maintenance, such as administration books, protocols, inspection records and managing documentations as well as storage inventories, purchase registries, lists of key suppliers, inventories, canteen menus and much more.

Another important resource conserved in former asylums' archives are photographic collections. Asylum staff made extensive and pioneering use of photography for a variety of purposes (Brookes 2011). Photography was used for advertisement purposes and professional photographers were often officially commissioned to realise photos of the asylum: panoramic vistas, pictures of splendid gardens and magnificent buildings and photos of interior spaces such as galleries, dormitories and infirmaries, depicting scenes of everyday life with patients ambling in flourished yards, entertaining in brightly lit halls and dining together in spacious canteens or depicting staff at work in clean and organised kitchens and medical cabinets. Such images were aimed at portraying the grandness of these medical spaces, representing and presenting the asylum as it was supposed to be: i.e. a great public infrastructure, a site of order and a model of efficient medical care. They were an important means of communication and promotion for the asylum towards policy makers and funders, the national and international community of fellow doctors, as well as the general public. As an example of these extensive photo and postcard collections, the former San Lazzaro asylum's archive, conserved at the *Biblioteca Scientifica Carlo Livi*, includes about 100,000 medical records and a photographic collection of over 1,500 pictures organised in hundreds of photographic albums, the majority of which are pictures of the asylum buildings, daily activities and patients' portraits.[4] Photography was also rapidly and extensively adopted in asylums as a medical tool to assist psychiatrists in the classification of illnesses and to document medical procedures and practices, pathologies and patients' development during the treatment. Pictures of patients were therefore often included in clinical logs and collected in thematic photo albums for documentary and study purposes. Although this was doubtlessly an innovative practice, as Barbara Brookes notes, photography eventually also 'became just one of the ways in which people were transformed into records for state purposes' (Brookes 2011: 32).

Along with books, texts and photographic collections, a large share of former asylums' archives is usually constituted by former patients' medical records and clinical logs. Once a person was admitted at the asylum, a patient casebook was created including their complete medical history. Casebooks usually included a patient's personal data: namely, date and place of their birth, ethnicity, origin and living address. It also included information on patients' social and economic status – typically their educational level, religion, civil status and profession – as well as annotations on patient's way of living, family and their social behaviours. Such notes were complemented by a clinical description of the patient upon hospital admission, noting reason for internment, a preliminary diagnosis, their physical and mental status, sometimes a picture and a brief inventory of clothes worn and personal belongings held at the moment of their internment. Asylum inmates were in fact usually obliged to wear the asylum's institutional clothing; toiletries and anything else needed for personal care and everyday activity was to be approved and/or provided by the asylum staff. As Nicole Baur and Joseph Melling, and Bronwyn Labrum separately point out in discussing the use medical and social meanings of clothing in 19th-century asylums: 'institutional clothing formed part of a hospital regimen of overt control, as well as meeting considerations of economy and employment' (Baur and Melling 2014: 152; Labrum 2011). Upon admission, patients' personal belongings and clothes were taken and packed away in appropriate storage – in Italian asylums, this was a specific building located nearby the asylum's main entrance and administration blocks, called *fagotteria*, literally 'the bundles storage-room'.

Casebooks were constantly updated throughout the patient's stay and, in cases of subsequent hospital admissions to the asylum, from their first arrival to the end of the stay – be it for final dismissal or death. Therefore, they also include observation notes by nurses and doctors on a patient's conduct during their interment, their physical and mental status and progresses, records of treatments and responses, medical documents and analysis and administrative documents such as letters of hospitalisation, dismissal, transfer to other pavilions or asylums or death certificate. In some cases, they also included not-strictly-medical documents, such as personal correspondence to and from relatives and friends, and between the doctor and the family members.

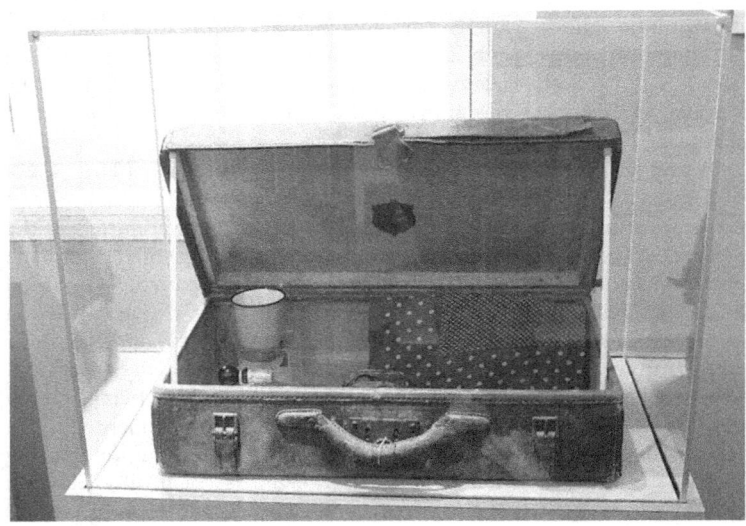

Image 2.1 The exhibition *The Lives They Left Behind* was on display at the *Museum of disABILITY History* in Buffalo until December 2020, when the museum definitively closed down.

The exhibition was based on a collection of over 400 patients' suitcases abandoned and found in the attic of the Willard Psychiatric Center when the institution closed in 1995. It is also a compelling example of the great outreach potential of such heritage of mental health produced by, within and around the asylum, and its capability to raise interest and to foster a debate about past and present approaches to mental health care among the general public. The suitcases were first discovered by staff members Beverly Courtwright and Lisa Hoffman, with Craig Williams, a *New York State Museum* curator, who were scouring the hospital premises 'trying to safeguard anything that might be worth keeping before the buildings were condemned' (Stastny and Penney 2008: 13). In 1999, Darby Penney, an American mental health worker, human rights activist and psychiatric survivor, who was working as director of Recipient Affairs at the New York State Office of Mental Health came to learn about the suitcases from Williams, who, four years before, had managed to move them into the museum's warehouse, despite the museum's scepticism on his intention to keep them all. Penney, with her colleague Peter Stastny, a psychiatrist and documentary filmmaker, and photographer Lisa Rinzler, started researching the life and stories of the 427 people who owned each of those suitcases. Their work resulted in an exhibition at the *New York State Museum* in 2004, attended by over 600,000 visitors; the exhibition subsequently travelled for 10 years across the United States, and was displayed in 30 venues in 11 different states, finally arriving at the *Museum of disABILITY History* in Buffalo in 2015. In December 2020 the *Museum of disABILITY History*, which has been closed to the public through the COVID-19 pandemic, has announced its permanent closure.

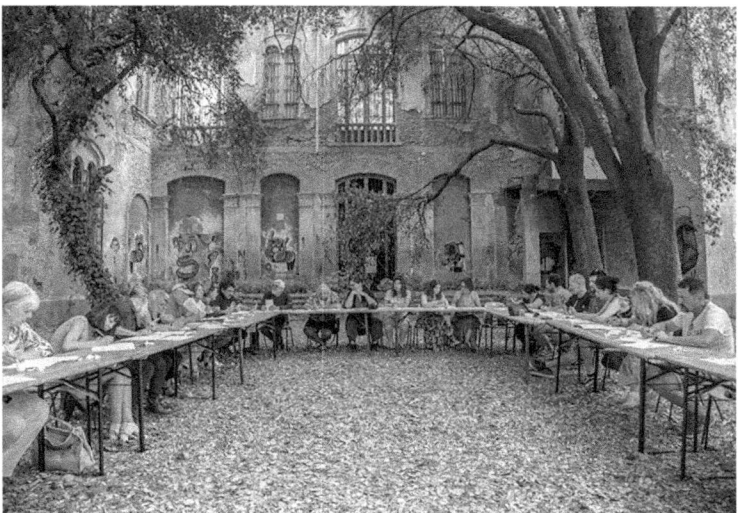

Image 2.2 Public art project *Corrispondenze Immaginarie* [Imaginary Correspondence] by Mariangela Capossela, Volterra 2022.

In 1983, Carmelo Pellicanò superintendent doctor at the Volterra Asylum during the transition years of the implementation of the hospital closure, published a book with his collaborators, Remigio Raimondi, Giuseppe Agrimi and Volfango Lusetti e Mauro Gallevi Cover titled *Corrispondenza negata: Epistolario della nave dei folli* (1889–1974) [*Denied Correspondence: Letters from the Ship of Fools* (1889–1974)]. The book collects a selection among the thousands of letters written from 1889 to 1974 by asylum patients to their loved ones outside the asylum but never sent and kept by the asylum in patients' medical records as evidence supporting their diagnosis. Drawing in this research and publication, in 2022, over 460 of these letters have been carefully hand rewritten by a group of participants and sent to patients' families as part of a public art project by the artist Mariangela Capossela titled C.I. *Corrispondenze Immaginarie*. © 2022 Corrispondenze Immaginarie.

Former asylums' medical collections and archives today constitute the oldest core of mind museums' collections. As we will see in this chapter, historical objects from asylums' psychiatric collections are invariably ever present in the display of each and every mind museum, becoming iconic objects of these exhibitions. Their preservation and study are at the roots of mind museums' birth and today they are key aspects of their work. After the closure of asylums, many former asylums' archives were conserved, wholesale or in part, by asylum and mind museums as part of their collections and then researched, deployed in educational activities of different kinds and exhibited in their display.[5] Whilst the historical origins of mind museums' collections lie in 19th-century asylum collecting practices, their development into public forms of display are to be found in the memorialisation endeavour and associated exhibition practices spurred by the deinstitutionalisation process and the closure of the asylum in the second half of the 20th century gave birth to asylum museums.

Saved and displayed: Asylum museums

As mentioned above, forms of collecting and display were common in the asylum; however, this mainly happened within asylum walls and institutional dynamics, not for public consumption, nor with any educational or didactic rationale, but chiefly for personal and institutional purposes. Still today, as Coleborne and Mackinnon articulate, many psychiatric asylum collections are difficult to access and research. Most of them are private, and very few are held by public museums or open to the general public, meaning they remain mostly 'inaccessible to the broader community now, as they once were when they were in use within psychiatric institutions' (Coleborne and MacKinnon 2011: 8). Mind museums constitute a major and radical change in this tradition of psychiatric collecting and display. To understand and appreciate the scope of this change, I will, here, culturally and politically frame it within the 'rupture' (Coleborne 2020) brought about by the deinstitutionalisation process and the associated 'revolts' (Crossley 2006).

As Catherine Coleborne articulates in her recent work *Why Talk About Madness* (2020), deinstitutionalisation has brought 'madness' to the fore of the public debate and has propelled a variety of new and previously unthinkable opportunities for the discussion and critique of mental health care within and beyond the medical sphere. It contributed to making mental health problems more visible in communities and no longer institutionally confined and secluded. At the same time, it has contributed the disclosure of some previously inaccessible resources that helped articulate and promote new discourses around mental health within the public sphere. Deinstitutionalisation was fundamentally an ideologically driven process, a cultural revolution as much as a medical reform, which created a breach in the narrative of mental health and made it possible to develop new ways to talk about mental health and its care, including within museums. At the same time, the closure of psychiatric asylums has set the very material condition for the birth of mind museums, by making available both historical collections and archives for them to be re-searched, studied and eventually displayed, as well as the physical spaces where these displays are located, namely former asylums' pavilions. In this context developed the very first forms of public exhibitions of stories and collections of mental health – asylum museums – which were, in effect, the first generation of mind museums.

The birth of asylum museums has been largely a bottom-up phenomenon carried out by members of those communities that felt themselves variously bound to the asylum, former nurses and doctors in particular. The loss of a sense of community and purpose that the closure of the asylum represented for these people and communities has thus often been accompanied by an upsurge of memorialisation instances, which would eventually lay the foundation for the birth of asylum museums and museums of mental health (Brüggemann and Schmid-Krebs 2007; Flis and Wright 2011; Guillemain 2013; Labrum 2011; Maj 2013). Not infrequently, once asylums started to be closed, relocated or downsized, individuals or groups of collectors – usually former doctors and nursing staff – compelled by the perceived urgency to document, save and preserve a past that was about to radically change, started to collect the material memory of the asylum. At first, such collecting was very spontaneous, unsystematic and characterised by a certain level of serendipity. It often took the form of hectic and frantic runs for salvaging whatever possible and considered worthy from decay, disposal and looting by rummaging in closed pavilions, abandoned doctor's offices and storages. Its aim was basically to retrieve and recover anything that could be found in a good state of preservation and that might be considered somehow meaningful and representative of the asylum life, for good or bad. Virtually all the curators and staff members working in contemporary asylum and mind museums I spoke with confirmed the crucial role of this spontaneous endeavour for the formation of the collections that their museums today conserve and display. Many of the museum staff were directly involved in these ventures. A sense of pride surfaces from their accounts for what is described as a somehow heroic and forward-looking endeavour, that is told as what made it possible to 'save this heritage' – as they say – and 'pass it on' to today's generations and those that will follow.

Some of the objects collected were retrieved from those historical medical collections assembled within the asylum during the 19th and the first half of the 20th century. However, more, newer and many ordinary objects were also collected, with a preference for objects connected to the asylum's material culture and daily life and activities. These typically included clothing items, like staff and patients' uniforms, shoes, aprons and other garments; everyday objects, such as crockery, linens, cutlery, dishes, jars, flatware, chamber pots, etc.; working tools, including woodwork tools, looms and gardening tools; sport equipment, boardgames and embroidering works. Tools and equipment for medical care were collected as well, most frequently syringes, test tubes, bandages and medical devices for physical restrain as straps, leather, nylon or vinyl waist belt and wrist cuff, and various types of straitjackets. Small pieces of furniture were also saved up, when possible, like barber chairs, sturdy hard wire beds, containment beds, desks, glass showcases, medication cabinets and glazed dressers. In some cases, whole room settings were recovered. Patient-made artifacts were also collected.[6] In most cases, such collecting practices also took place and continued outside of the asylum walls at a community level, through donations and minor acquisitions, with museum volunteers scouting among local people and other former staff member for asylums objects, pictures, documents and, more recently, by collecting oral histories.

Soon after, from the late 1970s and especially during the 1980s, asylum museums started to appear, frequently in disused former asylums buildings, now makeshift venues for the sheltering and exhibition of collections of objects that had been 'saved and displayed'. Asylum museums are often amateur museums. They are usually funded, designed and run by volunteers, many of whom were previously asylum employees. Asylum museums are generally small-scale and local museums, mostly subsisting on fundraising and volunteers work to survive. As might be expected, their opening hours are often limited, outreach through museum-produced communication is practically absent and usually only available in the local language. It is therefore very difficult to have a comprehensive picture of the state of the art of such museums. From the scarce information available and the limited literature focusing on them, it emerges, however, that there is a relatively large number of asylum and mental health museums across Western Europe, with many characteristic features in common.[7] Among them, the *Glenside Hospital Museum* (GHM) in the United Kingdom is a paradigmatic example.

GHM is located in the old chapel of the former Bristol Lunatic Asylum on Blackberry Hill in the suburb of Fishponds, northeast of Bristol, about 3 miles (5 km) from the city centre. As we can read on the museum website: 'the museum was founded by Dr Donal Early, a consultant psychiatrist at Glenside Hospital. Objects and documents were *saved and collected* from all corners of the building and beyond' (italics added, GHM website [Last Accessed, October 2022]). 'Since the mid-1950s – we learn from on-site informative material – staff members of Glenside Hospital have saved memorabilia typical of mental hospital life. This wonderful haphazard collection, added to by other hospitals and institutions, now constitutes the *Glenside Hospital Museum*, which aims to represent, warts and all, what hospital life was like for staff and patients in bygone days' (the informative material is signed: John Bartlett (chairman) Fishponds Local History Society, June 2001). From 1984, the GHM collection was displayed on a balcony in the dining room of the former asylum. In 1994, following the asylum closure and site conversion into a university campus,[8] the museum was moved into the former hospital's chapel, a grade II listed building given to the museum by the new site owner, the University of West of England, on a nominal rent. Volunteers were actively involved in works to convert the chapel into an exhibition space by 'scrubbing the floors, removing the boards from the windows, placing the exhibits on the pews' (GHM website [Last Accessed, October 2022]). In 2009, the museums closed for building repair works, and its main exhibition was renewed; designed and realised by volunteers, it remains mostly unchanged since 2010, when the museum reopened.

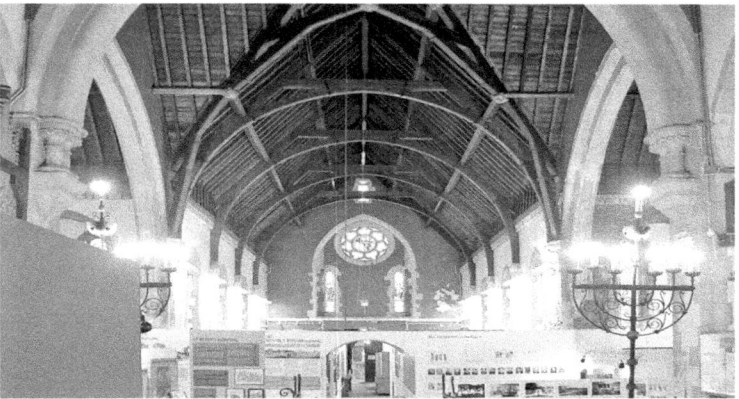

Image 2.3 The *Glenside Hospital Museum* (GHM) set up in the old chapel of the former Bristol Lunatic Asylum on Blackberry Hill, Fishponds, Bristol.
Photo by Francesca Lanz, July 2021.

The former chapel space hosting the museum is divided in three main areas. In the transept, in front of the entrance, there is the staff area, including an office space, a kitchenette and the front desk, which is also used to display publications, booklets, pamphlets and postcards about the museum (many of which are produced in-house). The choir stalls are occupied by an exhibition on the Stoke Park Hospitals for Learning Disabilities,[9] and other smaller temporary displays related to museum projects and activities. The altar space is a used as an archive-library. The main exhibition it is set up along the chapel's main nave. It focuses on the history of Glenside Hospital and the whole museum collection, except for very few objects, is on display here. The space of the main nave is divided into smaller exhibitions spaces by a continuous stud wall structure, consisting of white-painted plaster walls about 2.5 metres high. This forms rooms of a sort and serves as the physical support for exhibitions, incorporating wall-mounted display cases of different kinds and sizes.

The exhibition retraces the history of the asylum. The collection is displayed following a not entirely consistent chronological and thematic ordering criteria within a sequence of rooms disposed along a central corridor each of which focus on theme or an asylum space – the morgue, the hairdresser, nurse training, insulin therapy, etc. In some rooms, dioramas (full-size reconstructions populated by mannequins) are put side by side with glass display cases crowded with objects; on the walls are hung various historical documents (photos of the asylum, site plans, prints, portraits of former doctors and nurses, medical certificates, etc) and also information panels, labels and pre-spaced adhesive vinyl texts and graphics. The space is literally filled with informations, data, memories and memorabilia of the asylum. Because of the number and variety of objects and information presented, the mixed ordering criteria and the labyrinthine layout, the exhibition turns out to be quite overwhelming overall and occasionally confusing. The visitor is left with very little space – mental, emotional *and* physical – for appraising the meaning and stories beyond the objects and stories on display. Due to the crowded organisation of the space, objects tend to blur with one another, eventually diminishing any visual and storytelling potential they may have. At the same time, because of such visually and intellectually overpowering display, the visitor can also quickly forget about being in former asylum building – namely a chapel of a former asylum, which incidentally is relatively well-conserved overall, featuring several original features including the pulpit, the altar, the organ[10] and very interesting and meaningful stained glasses.

Although asylum museums' displays generally exhibit very rich collections and are based on sometime very accurate historical research – 'interesting' and 'informative' are the most recurrent adjectives used to describe the GHM by visitors,[11] they are in effect more a resource in its raw state than a 'sophisticated form of representation and communication that aims to present particular narratives or organisations of knowledge, or to create sensory environments and affective spaces that invite or impel visitors to respond in a certain way' (Whitehead 2016a: 2). Like the GHM, asylums' museums focus on the on the history of psychiatric institutions with key regard to the asylum where they are located and from which their collection originates from. The amount of objects on display is usually quite large, practically the whole collection: this not so much because of the lack of storage space as a consequence of the enthusiasm and attachment of those who set up the display to each and every piece of the collection. This, in most cases, has been physically assembled by the same volunteers running the museum and it often also includes some of their own personal memorabilia of the asylum and objects sourced in loan or as donation to the museum by family members, friends, former colleagues and members of the local communities. The collection is usually displayed following an institutional-history-based chronological

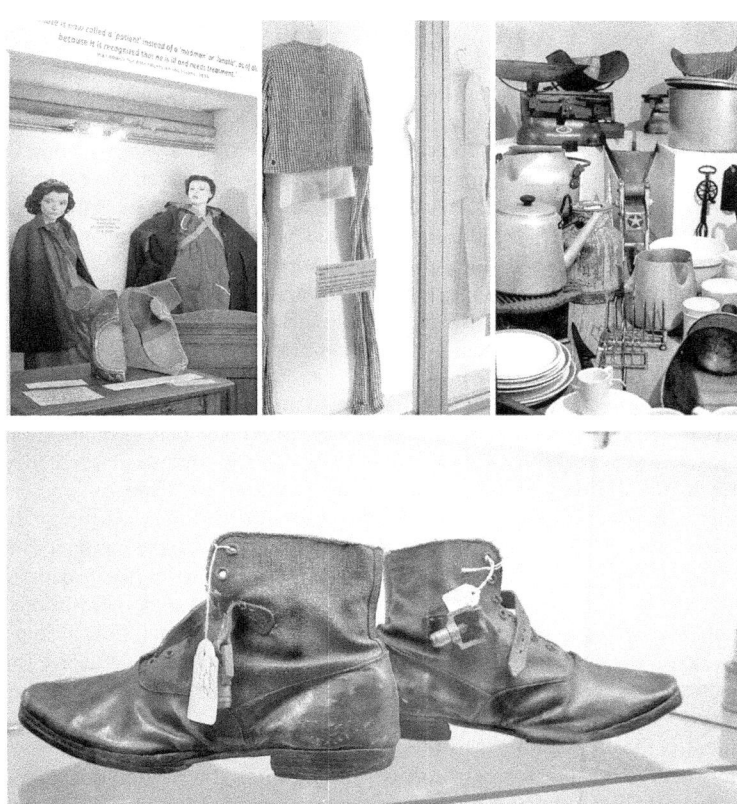

Image 2.4 Glenside Hospital Museum (GHM): On the left, diorama with mannequins wearing hospital uniforms in the section on 'Nurse Training'.
On the right, a pair of lockable boots on display in the section about 'Hospital Housekeeping'. When I visited the museum with the curator Stella Mann, she pointed me to these boots, which I did not notice at first. These are one of their favourite objects in the museum. She told me that the first time she saw them, she thought they were a sort of restraint tools; they made her think of heavy metal prisoner shackles and metal convict balls, as those you see in films. However, once she learned about their design was to avoid laces for patients' security, she started to look at them in a new way; they became to her an example of design for care, not for harm, as well as a symbol of the stereotypes we have about mental asylums as places of torture. These boots are Stella's memory anchor. A similar pair of boots are on display at the *Bethlem Museum of the Mind*; I noticed them only after having met Stella. On the bottom right one of memories shared by museum visitors shared in an designed space within the exhibition. The note reads: '1978. I remember the pride / worry at collecting my new striped student nurse uniform after completing

ordering with tens of exemplars of similar items literally crammed into display cases grouped thematically. In addition to a such a large amount of objects, the display usually includes an extremely rich and heterogenous informative apparatus consisting of labels, information panels of different sizes and types – comprising text, images and graphics – and hand-in information sheets, flyers, booklets and publications – many of which were written by volunteers themselves. The overall visual effect of these exhibitions is often quite striking, not least for the aesthetic impact of such forms of accumulation. However, this is mostly an incidental effect rather than a purposely deployed display strategy.

Asylum museums are in fact usually the result of a spontaneous acts of preservation and exhibition, often self-designed and sometimes even self-produced by part-time curators and the volunteers themselves with practically no funding nor professional standards of collecting, conservation or display and without any underlying museum strategy and mission other than saving and displaying asylum memorabilia. This has important consequences on both how these museums are and look, and what they mean. Firstly, they are often the result of an impulse towards memorialisation amongst members of communities in decline in an attempt to preserve a past, a vision of their own world and its daily life, routines and physical places, in a moment when they were about to radically change forever. As such, asylum museums can be quite nostalgic institutions. Furthermore, as visitors themselves are mainly local, including a large share of former staff members or family members, their reasons for visiting, their visiting experience and their accounts and reactions to it are very personal and often soaked with nostalgic feelings similar to those that boosted the establishment of the museum itself. Because of that, asylum museums, much like forms of collecting done within the asylum during the 19th and 20th centuries, retain an ambiguous identity somewhere in-between a public museum and a private collection of memorabilia assembled and displayed as a form of identity affirmation. A palpable tension emerges from their display between, on the one hand, such a nostalgic feeling, a celebrative reminiscence of a 'golden age of the asylum' and an evident place attachment and, on the other, a substantially evolutionary view of psychiatry, where the past of 'institutional psychiatry' is represented and rejected as dark, grim and abusive and the present

---

PTS (pre training school) – button from the neck down – and paper hat with 1 band (1 for 1st year). I sadly remember pts [patients] eating from the "pig bins", walking with trousers too short and buying one fag at a time from the hosp [hospital] shop. However I remember the grounds that staff + pt [patient] could sit in, the community which accepted and celebrated behaviour which was different from the "norm"' (Anonymous comment, GHM 'My Memory of the Asylum' display, n.d.) Photos by Francesca Lanz, July 2021.

is represented as revolutionary, humane and progressive. The past is located in a distant time, a 'then' separated from the deinstitutionalised 'now'. This is something that, as Bronwyn Labrum rightfully points out, 'allow[s] visitors to put exhibitions of madness and psychiatry firmly into the distant past, rather than seeing the continuities with the recent past or indeed with the present' (2011: 80).

A similar detachment and dystopia also characterise asylum museums' exhibition design. This is often quite simple and amatorial – in many cases, self-design and even self-realised consisting of stud walls and stand-alone glass cabinets. ECT machines, lobotomy kits, strait-jackets and tools for mechanical restraint – notably fetters and shackles – are ever present objects. Mannequins wearing original and uniforms are also recurrent as well as more or less historically accurate full-scale reconstructions of original asylums spaces and ambiances – typically the padded cell, the inmate rooms, the old pharmacy and the doctor's cabinet. Above all, their exhibition design is generally unresponsive and indifferent to the context where is it set up. Not only does the creation of these museums rarely involve any architectural interventions onto the pre-existing fabric other than the bare minimum needed to adapt the space for the new use, but in no case does it attempt to establish a dialogue with the context – the (former) asylum out there. Emblematically full rooms and asylum spaces are reconstructed using leftover furniture or replicas, while the fact that the museum is actually located within an 'original' space itself is somehow ignored. As a result, the context is silenced, and the display is separated both aesthetically and in terms of its contents and focus from its exhibition environment, completely overlooking its actual potential and possible contribution to the museum story-telling and meaning making.

In many regards, asylum museums are often somehow 'voyeuristic' not only in their exhibition design and techniques but also in their 'insistence that the history of madness is one of violence and trauma' (Flis and Wright 2011: 107; Labrum 2011; Moon et al. 2015: 70–85). Furthermore, precisely because (as noted earlier) they are first and foremost about the staff and the place, the patient is in effect absent, mute and invisible in the collections as much as in their display. The patients are either 'subsumed within their environment [...] secondary figures [whose] material culture forms a subset of this displayed' (Labrum 2011: 71, 79), or implicitly 'neglected' and 'victimised' (Flis and Wright 2011: 107). Bronwyn Labrum's (2011) description of a display of an isolation cell and empty wardrobes at the small *Kenmore Hospital Museum* in Goulburn Australia is emblematic as much as the display of chain and fetters at *Museo di San Servolo* in Venice Italy represented in the images below. This voyeuristic drift, not only disempowers the patients, but also, although unintentionally, plays out an imaginary one that resonates with a popular culture of the asylum as a 'place of horror'. Added to this, the fact that such exhibitions are often set up pavilions, located in semi-deserted former asylum sites, often partially decaying, and such exhibitionary environments effectively create an aura of secrecy and dread. This revives in people's minds grim visual imaginaries, tapped into a diffused visual culture of the asylum that often tend to blur together madhouses, asylums and mental hospitals and mingling their horrors and mistakes with those of other 20th-century total institutions as prisons and workhouses up to concentration camps and other sites of confinement, internment and torture.[12]

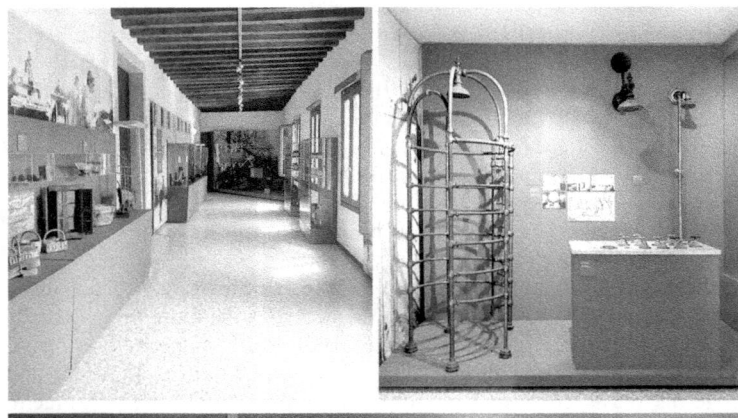

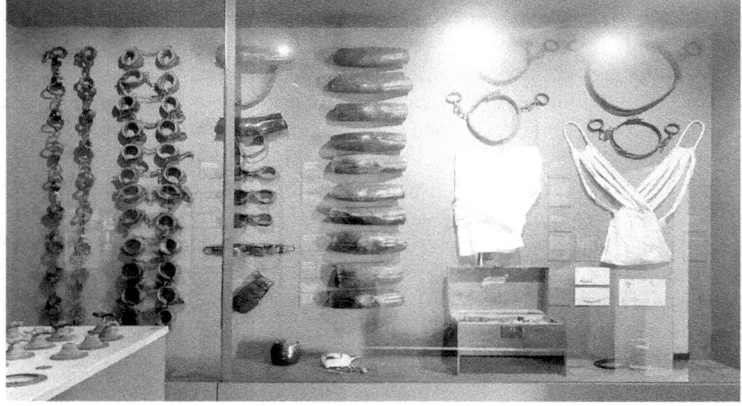

Image 2.5 Museo del Manicomio di San Servolo – La Follia reclusa, Venice, Italy.
The first section of the permanent exhibition is devoted to 'Therapies': hydrotherapies, ergotherapy, drug therapy, electroconvulsive therapy and shock therapies, and musicotherapy. Despite the exhibition's thematic arrangement, each section follows

Because of all that, these museums, with their 'emphasis on relics as opposed to a focus on systems of care and on caring itself' (Moon et al. 2015: 82) , their 'displays of electro-shock machines and lobotomy tools' and full-scale reconstructions and evocative environments, may paradoxically risk ending up reinforcing stereotypes about the asylum and mental health care although the feelings of community attachment they embody would have a potential to mollify, if not overcome, the impact of stigma attached to these former asylum and mental health care more broadly. Nonetheless, these museums have to be credited with the merit of opening up psychiatric collections and the asylum for the first time to the general public and, in doing so, of having unlocked the potential of the heritage of mental health. Asylum museums have made accessible a material culture and memories previously concealed almost privately within the asylum and by individuals. They, and the commemoration practices they represent, offer new forms and opportunities of public engagement with mental health issues that have the potential to create new narratives tapped into the heritage of mental health they convey. All that is taken over and capitalised upon by a new generation of museums, which I call mind museums.

A new generation of museums

Mind museums are young, scarce in number and relatively small institutions. Most of them were opened in the first decades of the 2000s. Examples

---

a chronological ordering criterion, meaning the therapies are presented in order of their advent in the asylum. The 'Therapies' section develops along a long corridor: there are windows facing the internal yard on one side, display pedestals and glass cases on the opposite one and a grand piano at the end of the corridor. The space is neat and bright: a few selected objects are displayed against a backdrop of full-scale reproductions of historical pictures, and the main colour of the exhibition is a sober deep mid-blue. Soon after the section's entrance, on the left, there is a small room where both hydrotherapy and restraint devices are together on display, perhaps for chronological reasons. The room has no windows, and the exhibition apparatus consists of a bright-red stud-wall structure that upholsters two of the four walls and embeds a floor-to-ceiling glass display case and a pedestal. In the glass, case is hung tens of mechanical restraint tools – including chains, wrist fetters, handcuffs, ankles blockers, iron belts – and a straitjacket, as well as a supporting smock used for bath-tube therapies, an insufflator, an inhalator and a 19th-century first-aid resuscitating kit. On the pedestal there is a shower with a cage, two other types of showers and a water valve station controlling different taps and various water temperatures. The juxtaposition of such different objects, from different ages and used for different purposes, is very confusing. Complicit the dramatic light spots, and the small, windowless bright-red painted room, it is quite easy to slip into nightmarish imaginaries and misinterpret objects: the smock becomes another straitjacket, the shower a medieval cage, the resuscitating kits and the valve station, strange unknown torture instruments. Photos by Francesca Lanz, July 2021.

include three Italian museums: The *Museo di Storia della Psichiatria*, opened in 2006 in the Lombroso pavilion at the former San Lazzaro mental asylum in Reggio Emilia (Lanz and Montanari 2022; Lanz 2020; Grassi et al. 2013; Tagliabue 2013); the MAPP, *Museo di Arte Paolo Pini*, located on the ground of the former Mental Hospital Paolo Pini in Milan, which started its activities in 1995 (Breckner et al. 2004); and the *Museo Laboratorio della Mente* in Rome, hosted in pavilion N°. 06 at the former mental hospital Santa Maria della Pietà in Rome, opened in 2008 and currently closed for a major renovation (Aglieri Rinella 2013; Boyd and Hughes 2020: 23–50; Cirifino et al. 2011; Fusco et al. 2017; 2019; Mandelli 2019; Martelli et al. 2013; Museo Laboratorio della Mente and Studio Azzurro 2019; Valentini 2017). Other European examples of mind museums are the *Bethlem Museum of the Mind*, opened in 2015 in the former administration block of the still-working Bethlem Royal Hospital in Beckenham, near London (Jay 2016); the *Dr Guislain Museum* in Gent, firstly opened in 1986 in the premise of the oldest Belgium asylum and renovated several times, most recently in 2019 (Unhinged 2019); and the *Museum of the Mind – Museum van de Geest* in the Netherlands, which comprises two venues: the *Museum of the Mind | Outsider Art* hosted at the *Hermitage Amsterdam* since 2016, and the *Museum of the Mind | Dolhuys,* located in a former leper, pauper hospital and madhouse in Haarlem, reopened after a restoration of its hosting building and redesign of its exhibition in 2021.

As mentioned, when it comes to the politics of mental health and the landscape of mental health heritage, the Italian context is both unique and paradigmatic. Italy not only fully embraced and further developed ideas and approaches promoted by the antipsychiatric movement that was thriving across Europe in the 1950s but it is the country that, more than any other, pushed forward the deinstitutionalisation process, leading to the closure of all mental hospitals of any kind, including forensic ones. Furthermore, although most of them are currently in a state of abandonment and total or partial disuse, there is a relatively high number of still-standing historical former asylum architectural complexes across Italy compared to other countries, such as the United Kingdom, where the great majority of them have been either demolished or sold and repurposed – in most cases for residential development. The simple presence of such large, complex and layered architectural assets constitutes a challenge, but it also offers remarkable opportunities and space for experimentation and the implementation of interventions aimed at their valorisation and preservation through their reuse, notably here their musealisation. Some of these reuse interventions explore and provide seminal examples of how these sites may be preserved and valorised, respecting the multiple, and sometimes conflicting 'traces' (Anderson 2021) that superimpose on these sites, while at the same time enabling their reappropriation by new and evolving communities.

Among these, the *Museo Laboratorio della Mente* is one of the very first and most pioneering mind museum in the contemporary international scene. Inaugurated in 2008, the *Museo Laboratorio della Mente* originates from a previous exhibition titled *La Linea d'Ombra: l'assistenza psichiatrica a Roma dal XVI al XX secolo* [*The Shadow Line; Psychiatric Care in Rome from XVI to XX Century*] set up in the nineties on the ground floor of a disused pavilion of the former asylum Santa Maria della Pietà. The Santa Maria della Pietà was Rome's main mental asylum, purposely built in the early 20th century (1909–1924) in the Monte Mario outskirt neighbour-hood.[13] At the time of its construction, it represented a pioneering example and a reference model for its innovative design. However, originally planned to host 1,000 patients, it soon overcrowded, reaching up to over 3,500 patients. As other asylums across the country, it was officially closed in 1978, following the ratification of the Basaglia Law, with the last patients finally dismissed in 1999. The exhibition *La Linea d'Ombra* was opened in 1995; conceived and developed within the cultural context of the Italian social and radical psychiatric movement, it was designed and set up by former asylum staff members led by Dr Pompeo Martelli (a therapist working at the Santa Maria della Pietà in those years) at a moment of radical change and break with asylum institutional past with the chief aim to 'describe the life in the asylum' to a public who were mostly unaware of it (Fusco et al. 2017: 69).

La Linea d'Ombra primarily consisted of a series of full-scale reconstruc-tions of certain rooms and spaces of the asylum and displaying original furniture and objects retrieved from the asylum stores. In this form, it fitted the description of an asylum museum as outlined in the preceding chapter. After an update and extension in 2000, the exhibition was eventually closed to reopen in a radically renewed form in 2008 on the same site – the pavilio no. 6 of the Santa Maria della Pietà former asylum, but with the new name: *Museo Laboratorio della Mente*. Still under the scientific curatorship of the museum founder and director Dr Pompeo Martelli, the driving idea beyond such radical renewal was to evolve the exhibition from a 'collection' to a 'narration' (Martelli 2019: 13) and to shift its focus from asylum history to mental health debate. Although part of the new museum's scope has in effect remained that of documenting the history of asylum institutions, the *Museo Laboratorio della Mente* substantially differs from its previous incarnation, for it has openly and consciously taken on as its core mission 'to develop a continuous reflection on the paradigm health/illness, on ideas of otherness, on social inclusion, on the politics of care and culture and community engagement' (MLM website [accessed October 2022]). To do that, a key role has been entrusted to its new exhibition, titled *Da Vicino Nessuno è Normale* [*Up Close Nobody is Normal*], designed by Studio Azzurro. Studio Azzurro is a renowned Italian group of multimedia artists experienced in the development of exhibitions based on new technologies and what they termed 'sensible ambiances' and 'narrative museums' (Cirifino et al. 2011; Valentini 2017). *Da Vicino Nessuno è Normale* features objects from the museum collection, historical documents, photographs and patients' medical cases and artworks, complemented by audio and video documentaries and a few information panels and synthetic labels. First and foremost, however, the exhibition was conceived as, and designed to be, a 'strong emotional experience' aimed at fostering understanding but not pity, spurring empathy and through that encouraging reflection on the nature of madness and how it was, and is, cured and perceived in contemporary society (Cirifino et al. 2011: 133).

The exhibition comprises 15 interactive installations, organised into 6 thematic sections, which the visitor is obliged to experience within a single predetermined path. These are: 'Entering Out, Exiting In', about the internment experience; 'Ways of Feeling', on perceptive alterations; 'Portraits', focusing on the representation of asylum's inmates; 'Houses of the Body', on bodily gestures, 'Inventors of Worlds', displaying artworks from two former inmates – one of which is Oreste Nannetti, who had been hospitalised for a short period in Rome before moving to Volterra; 'The Closed Institutions', about asylum institution violence and its impact on patients and staff lives; and 'The Factory of Change', on the history of the deinstitutionalisation movement in Italy. Two displays from the original exhibition *La Linea D'Ombra* – namely a room with a containment bed, that is a bed with strap restraints, and a medical office – conclude the visit. By making use of video projections, sounds, movement sensors and touch-sensitive screens, each installation offers an interactive, multi-sensorial, immersive experience where the visitor must touch and move to access information, which is often in the form of stories and witnesses. This requires the visitor to listen and pay attention. The visitor path develops on the ground floor of the pavilion, unfolding counterclockwise around a semi-transparent acrylic wall, structuring the visiting path and symbolising the separating and dividing logic of the asylum institution.[14] While considerable attention and effort has been put into the design of the exhibition, few changes have been made to the built fabric of the former asylum pavilion housing it, other than the minimum needed to turn it into a museum – namely the creation of a reception area with an office.

The *Museo Laboratorio della Mente* is today internationally considered a 'best practice' example among mental health cultural institutions and the wider museum community. Its award-winning exhibition has become widely famous for its pioneering use of new technologies and its poetic interactivity, often mentioned as one of the finest examples of Studio Azzuro museum design practices. Since 2008, the museum has attracted several sources of funding that have been used to support projects and collaborations of different kinds aimed at enlarging and updating its cultural offers. Among these, it promoted travelling exhibitions, artist in residency projects, art installations and a rich outreach and didactic programme (Museo Laboratorio della Mente and Studio Azzurro 2019). In 2011, a new display by Studio Azzurro, named *Portatori di Storie* [Bearers of Stories], temporarily hosted in the historical hospital library, was inaugurated (UOS Centro Studi e Ricerche ASL Roma e Studio Azzurro 2012). In 2021, the museum also opened a new site-specific installation titled *Ricordare il Futuro* [Remembering the Future]. The installation is set up in the former mental hospital archive and was realised by Blue Cinema TV using cinematic hologram technology to interactively allow visitors to browse and access medical records from the archive. In recent years, the museum has also started to increasingly work in context, to valorise the former asylum parkland and reweave it into the museum and the museum with the site's memories, histories and traces. This has been done mainly by promoting a series of site-specific art installations and place-based projects. In 2022, the *Museo Laboratorio della Mente* closed for a major refurbishment that will involve updating its exhibitions and the extension of the museum (mentioned earlier) to occupy the second floor of the pavilion, which will be restored and turned into a new exhibition space.

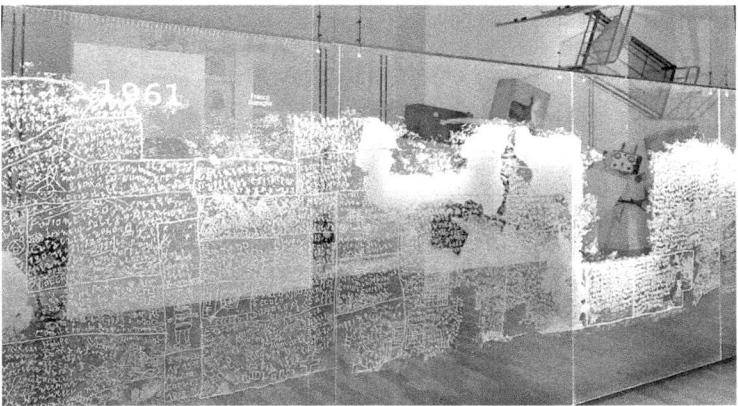

Image 2.6 The *Museo Laboratorio della Mente*, hosted at the pavilion No. 6 of the former psychiatric Hospital Santa Maria della Pietá in Rome, Italy.
View of the glass wall organising the exhibition and featuring NOF4 graffiti. Photo by Francesca Lanz, December 2019.

Along with this example from Rome, the *Bethlem Museum of the Mind* is the other most renowned example of a mind museum (Jay 2016). The *Bethlem Museum of the Mind* is located within the estate of the still-running

Bethlem Royal Hospital; the fourth incarnation of the Bethlem asylum is in Monks Orchard, Beckenham, about 20 kilometres south from London. The Bethlem asylum was originally founded in 1247 by Simon FitzMary and already in the 15th century it specialised in curing the 'insane' (Andrews et al. 1998). In 1676, the hospital moved from its original location, the St Mary priory in Bishopgate, into a new purpose-built facility in Moorfields. This was a large and impressive building, designed by the architect Robert Hooke. The building was further enlarged in the 18th century and was used until the early 19th century, hosting over 100 inmates and becoming widely (in)famous across the nation. In 1815, due to the building's severe state of disrepair and neglect, and following several scandals concerning patients' conditions, the Bethlem hospital was moved to a new venue built in St George's Field in Southwark – today, hosting the Imperial War Museum. A new hospital complex was built for Bethlem in the early 20th century in its current location, Monks Orchard, south of London. The hospital, inaugurated in 1930, was the first in England to adopt a 'villa' model, consisting of different independent units located within an extensive parkland of over 200 acres. Today, this is open to the public, who can walk, run and exercise on the grounds of the hospital, or explore them following specific walking trails.

There has been a museum at Bethlem Royal Hospital since 1970, only small and initially hosted in a container, it served more as a makeshift storage and an archive than as an exhibition space. The museum was open to the public on weekdays and mainly displayed items from the museum's art collection. In 2015, the museum, renamed *Bethlem Museum of the Mind,* opened with a new exhibition in its new venue, the former hospital's administration block, a two-storey Art Deco building, which the museum shares with the *Bethlem Gallery,* an artist-led team art gallery established in 1997, providing a professional space for high-quality artwork and a supportive artist-focused environment. The building has been restored and purposely refurbished to be reused as a museum, including exhibition spaces for the museum and the Bethlem gallery, an art workshop as well as the needed facilities and complementary spaces, from a reception desk and a book shop to offices, toilets and lockers. The museum exhibition spaces are on the first floor, reached through the main central double-ramp art deco staircase, now flanked by the two statues known as 'Raving and Melancholy', realised in the 17th century by a Danish sculptor, Caius Cibber, for the gates of the Bethlem hospital in Moorfields. On the first floor, on the two sides of the hospital boardroom, restored and conserved as it was, there are two symmetric exhibition rooms: one is used for temporary exhibitions and the other hosts the permanent display of the museum. They are relatively small white-painted, with a few windows blinded by white panel curtains, a spotlight rail system on the ceiling and a wooden parquet floor; both rooms feature a outward projecting extension on one corner. Upon entering in such spaces, one could easily forget where they are, for the space looks and feels like a generic museum gallery characterised by a bright and neutral palette, with white and orange as the master colours and a natural durmast oak wood as the main material, used both for floors and the bespoke display apparatus and cases.

The museum main exhibition, as we can read on the welcoming panel, 'explores Bethlem's controversial and often misunderstood history through the lens of mental health issues which are as relevant today as they were in the past. It is intended to provide a starting point for discussion, debate and reflection'. The museum's main display and rich programme of temporary exhibitions are in fact less about the history of the hospital and more about raising questions and challenging assumptions about what mental health is. This is done in a discreet and sensible way, allowing different visitors to engage at different levels with the display and leaving a remarkable level for individual interpretation and reflection. The exhibition is dense but not crowded, featuring a selection of historical and more contemporary objects from the museum collection, textual resources, documents and historical photograph from the archives, together with a selection of former patients' and contemporary artworks and a few interactive displays. Although there is not a prefixed visiting path – the display is not chronological but thematically organised – the visitor is encouraged to cover the exhibition in a clockwise sense. This is organised in three thematic sections arranged around a central large wall-size double-faced display case that create a central square shape space, furnished with a leather sofa where visitors can

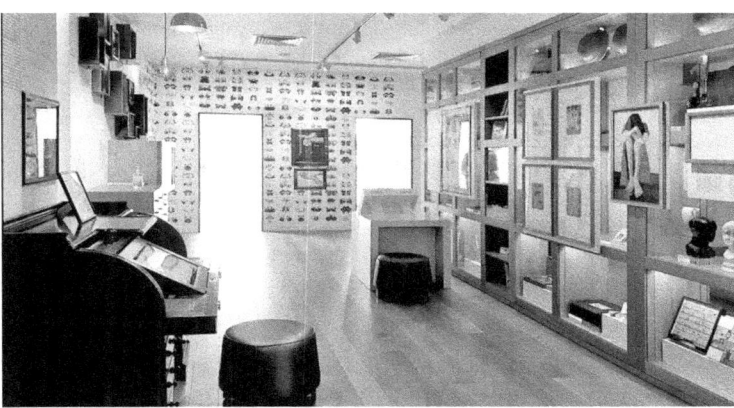

Image 2.7 The *Bethlem Museum of the Mind*, at the Bethlem Royal Hospital in Beckenham.
View of the first exhibition section on 'Labelling and Diagnosis'. Photo by Francesca Lanz July 2021.

sit and consult additional informative material and have a break from the visit at any time they may feel the need to do so. Each section is titled with an antithetic words-pair effectively introducing its focus in an already open and inquiring way: 'Labelling and Diagnosis', 'Freedom and Constraint' and 'Heal or Harm'.

A quite different type of mind museum is represent by the *Dr. Guislain Museum*. The museum, funded in 1986 by René Stockman, the museum's current curator and the Superior General of the Brothers of Charity, who was at that time also the Dr. Guislain Psychiatric Centre's general director. Today, the *Dr. Guislain Museum* has a hybrid identity somewhere in between a mind museum and a contemporary art gallery (*Unhinged* 2019). At the time of writing, its long-term exhibition *Unhinged*,[15] exhibits 'unique pieces alternate with compelling anecdotes, big theories with hidden testimonies' in line with the museum's intention to 'emphasise the acute importance of mental health today' (from the exhibition opening panel, July 2022). The exhibition is organised into five themes: 'Body and Mind', 'Classification', 'Architecture', 'Imagination and Power' and 'Powerlessness', the oldest item on display dating back to the 17th century and the most recent to 2017. Some of them are on loan from other, mainly private, Belgium-based collections, but the majority are part of *Dr. Guislain Museum*'s collection. Historical medical objects, books and documents from the asylum, together with older and contemporary artworks, mostly outsider art and art brute, are displayed with the declared aim to 'analyse that "other" that disturbs as well as fascinates' and raise the question 'where the does the norm end and chaos begin?' (from the exhibition opening panel, July 2022). At the time, I am writing, *Unhinged* flows almost with no interruption of any sort into the exhibition *Recovery Pathway*, the result of a 2019 participatory photovoice project in which eight women describe their daily life and their recovery processes in relation to 'illegal substance (ab) use' through a series of photographs.

A key question, implicit but underpinning the whole museum display, concerns contemporary medical approaches to mental health treatment. In particular, it questions the turn in Belgium's mental health politics during the early 2000s towards a community-based psychiatric care model. It does this, not by disapproving but rather by advocating for support and accountability in the care, support and assistance of those suffering from psychiatric vulnerability. It unsettlingly asks: '[T]here are also less visible forms of power like authoritative theories, common therapies and diagnoses. How do we recognise the power dynamics at a time of socialisation of health care? Do we cast a critical eye on psychiatry and the life in institutions or is it better to look at the words and images that surround us each day?' (from the panel 'Power and Powerlessness').

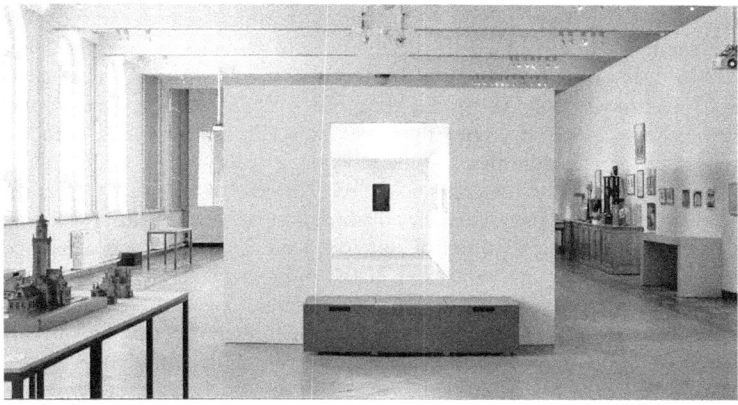

Image 2.8 The *Dr. Guislain Museum*, view of the current exhibition *Unhinged*.
Photo by Francesca Lanz, June 2022.

Finally, another different, somehow exceptional yet very telling example
of what a mind museum can be is offered by the MAPP – *Museo D'Arte
Paolo Pini* in Milan. The Paolo Pini psychiatric hospital was also officially
closed in 1978, but, like many other former asylums across the country, its
closure took years to be implemented and the last patients were dismissed in
the late 1990s. The architectural and functional evolution of the Paolo Pini
asylum is particularly complex and stratified because of the considerable
size of the site and its relatively central location in one of the biggest Italian
cities. Built in Affori, a suburban neighbourhood of Milan in the 1920s, the
asylum complex was enlarged, modified and upgraded throughout its entire
life span up until its dismissal and reuse, which, unlike most other cases, has
happened almost without any discontinuity, although in a rather scattered
and uncoordinated way (Breckner et al. 2004).

MAPP is a contemporary art gallery, an open-air museum and a
psychiatric day-centre promoting art therapy and running art-based
projects and artistic workshops targeted at people suffering from mental
health issues as part of their therapeutic treatment and recovery. The
project for the *MAPP* can be traced back to 1993 from an idea by Teresa
Melorio, a practising psychiatrist working at the Paolo Pini Hospital,
and Enza Baccei, a psychotherapist, with the artistic direction of Marco
Menguzzo. The initiative was undertaken in collaboration with the
Department of Mental Health at Hospital Niguarda Ca' Granda and in
conjunction with several prominent Milan-based art galleries. In 1995
Melorio and Baccei also founded the nongovernamental organisation
ARCA – *Associazione per il Recupero della Creatività Artistica e la*

Riabilitazione Psicosociale (Association for the Recovery of Art Creativity and Psych-social Rehabilitation); which is today responsible for running the museum and the therapeutic activities it promotes. The MAPP was officially recognized by Regione Lombardia as a museum in 2007. Its growing collection today comprises over 150 site-specific art works realised since 1993 by more than 140 artists in collaboration with the hospital's patients on the asylum pavilions' walls, and a collection of artworks realised within the so-called *Botteghe d'arte* – art therapy workshops – involving an artistic collaboration between artists and service users to co-produce artworks of different kinds. Artworks are conserved and exhibited with a rota system in the museum gallery located on the ground floor of pavilion N°. 7, where a number of workshop spaces have been set up in the former patients' rooms. The museum is open daily during the week, it organises site tours for the general public and schools guided by the MAPP's Divulgatori d'Arte – service users taking part in the *Botteghe d'Arte* and trained as cultural mediators and museum guides.

Today, the former Paolo Pini site and buildings host a large variety of functions and activities, some of which are related with the national health system, but also including various cultural associations, charities and NGOs. Among them is *Il Giardino degli Aromi Onlus* [The Garden of Aromas], founded in 2003 by a group of women with expertise in growing vegetables, culinary herbs and spices and medicinal herbs, with the mission to provide support for the social re-integration of vulnerable people, immigrants and asylum seekers through gardening-based activities. Another NGO on the site is Olinda Onlus. Olinda is a social enterprise and a collective project born in the early 1990s under the initiative of Rosita Volani, its artistic director, and the Swiss social entrepreneur and psychiatrist Thomas Emmenegger, *Olinda*'s founding president. The driving idea beyond the Olinda project is, as declared on their website, to explore 'how social inclusion and mental health can be pursued in urban suburbs? How can the space of exclusions be woven into the places of life, and how can health and social places and practices be intertwined with cultural places and practices? How can the heritage of the deinstitutionalisation experience be harvested and reinterpreted in an original way? How can we avoid recreating ghettoes?' (Olinda Website [Accessed October 2022]). Since its establishment, Olinda has been promoting a wide array of place-based events, activities and projects aimed at promoting the social inclusion of people suffering with mental health problems. It organises a yearly cultural and art festival named *Da Vicino Nessuno è Normale* [Up Close Nobody is Normal] and manages catering activities, a bistro, a theatre and a hostel. The hostel, located in a former asylum pavilion, experiments with forms of mixed hospitality by hosting tourists and housing former asylum residents with the active participation of service users in recovery as volunteers.

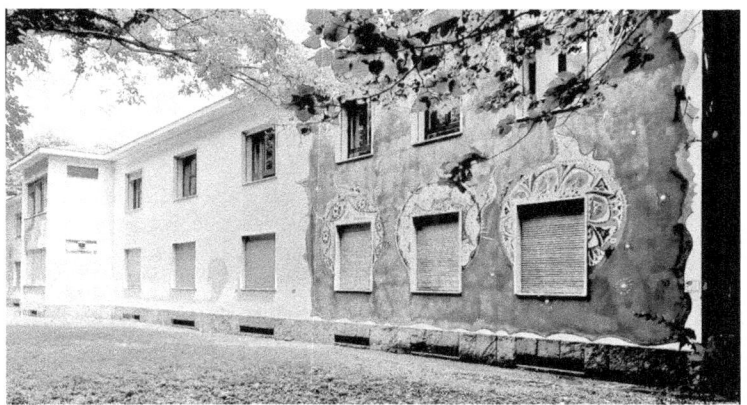

Image 2.9 The MAPP *Museo d'Arte Paolo Pini*, in the former Paolo Pini Psychiatric hospital in Milan.
Site-specific artwork by Riccardo Gusmaroli, 1995, murales with acrylic paint, Pavilion no. 07 – exterior.

From memorabilia display to museum laboratories

In their sheer diversity, the museums and experiences discussed previously are representative of the evolution of asylum museums into something new, which I call a 'mind museum'. A mind museum is a museum hosted in the disused spaces of a former mental asylum, which exhibitions focus on the history of its premise and mental health treatment. However, differently from asylum museums, a mind museum is not solely or chiefly a museum of social history or a museum of the history of psychiatry, nor is it simply is a former asylum building restored and conserved as a museum of itself. Rather, it is a site-specific and place-based cultural institution whose work and displays primarily pursue a mission to promote awareness about mental health care and to contribute to dismantling stigma and stereotypes surrounding mental health. It is difficult to draw a line between this definition of 'mind museums' and what has been previously described as an asylum museum. In many regards, mind museums are in fact an evolution of asylum museums. Some of them were actually established as an asylum museum; this is the case, for example, of the *Museo Laboratorio della Mente* in Rome or the *Bethlem Museum of Mind* in London. Others, however, are much newer, such as the *Museo di Storia della Psichiatria* in Reggio Emilia that will be discussed in detail in the following pages. Either way, asylum museums and mind museums do share some key characterising traits, notably the origin and nature of their collections and the fact that they are situated in a former asylum. Nonetheless, mind museums also differ markedly from any other previous forms of display and representations of the histories, stories, and the material culture of mental health in many aspects, including their size, their collecting and curatorial practices, collections management and display practices and exhibition design.

Firstly, compared to asylum museums, mind museums have done a significant scale-up. This is evident in the increased variety, number and ambition of the activities promoted by these museums, which play a crucial role in making mind museums more far-reaching in both their cultural relevance and outreach potential than asylum museums. Although the number of mind museum visitors is relatively small compared to other more established museums, this number is in fact significantly greater than the one of asylum museums. As an example, in 2018–2019, the *Bethlem Museum of the Mind* had an average of 10,000 visitors per year, compared to about 500 people visiting the GHM.[16] Furthermore, many mind museums have been able in a relatively short time to establish diffuse connections and networks at a regional, national and sometimes international level with diverse institutions, including other museums, libraries, archives, heritage trusts and networks, as well as NGOs, local health authorities, schools, universities and research centres. Being a part of cultural networks expose mind museums to broader cultural contexts and debate, facilitating enriching exchanges of ideas and enabling easier access to funding. Mind museums also exceed asylum museums in terms of their budget. In most cases, their birth is triggered by an initial one-off funding injection, after which all of them have proven thus far capable of catalysing interest and, with that, further economic support. As may be expected, the availability of funds has key consequences for their growth: supporting active collecting and the implementation of educational programmes, and the development of exhibitions and outreach projects.

The *Museo Laboratorio della Mente* is a paradigmatic example of this. Since its creation in 2008, it has garnered a very good national and international reputation with a steadily growing number of visitors. The museum has been awarded several prizes, including ICOM Italy 2010 Museum of the Year 'for its innovation and attractiveness in its relationship with the public' and in the past 15 years it has established a large network of collaborations with schools, university research centres, cultural institutions and national and international museums, recently becoming one of the funders and key promoters of the network *Mente in Rete*. The *Museo Laboratorio della Mente* is today also well-known amongst scholars and museums experts, featuring as a case study in a number of scholarly publications in Italian and English (Aglieri Rinella 2013; Boyd and Hughes 2020: 23–50; Cirifino et al. 2011; 2019; Fusco et al. 2017; 2019; Mandelli 2019; Martelli et al. 2013; Museo Laboratorio della Mente and Studio

Azzurro 2019). In this time, the museum has also been able to attract several national and international funding awards, most recently including a national public grant of 700,000 euros for the project *Portatori Sani di Diversitá* [Healthy Carriers of Diversity], involving the restoration and refurbishment of the second floor of the museum pavilion and the update and extension of its permanent exhibition.

However, what truly distinguishes mind museums from previous mental health and asylum museums is not merely their scale but, first and foremost, the heightening of their actual and desired societal impact and how that reflects in an expanded mission for such museums. Like asylum museums, mind museums also are products of deinstitutionalisation, but not so much in material terms as in their raison d'être and ambitions. Deinstitutionalisation and the core ideology beyond it, were as much about closing the asylum as it was about *opening it up* both literally and metaphorically: opening the asylum to society and communities to otherness, psychiatric practices and debate to other disciplines and voices – notably those of patients. They questioned the status quo and challenged the often exclusive or hierarchical conversations that have characterised the areas of mental health in the past to ensure that those who struggle with mental health become visible and their voices heard. These same ideals are driving elements in the project of mind museums and strongly resonate in their mission, displays and work.

The origins of many mind museums are indeed found in the aftermath of deinstitutionalization. Their development and emergence owe much to the antipsychiatric movements and deinstitutionalization ideologies, as well as to the vision and cultural entrepreneurship of individuals actively involved in asylum reforms of the time.[17] However, while the same can be said about asylum museums, crucially unlike them, mind museums are not the outcome of a spontaneous and conservation endeavour of a group of enthusiasts animated by the aim of saving and displaying memorabilia and the material culture of the asylum. Instead, they are the result of a well-structured all-round cultural project, which draws on the insights and knowledge of those people who have first promoted their creation, yet expanded and enriched in time and conjoined with other specific and professional museum skills. Such project revolves around a critical reflection on the past and present politics of mental health care, which future directions it aims help informing. Mind museums in fact seek to be more than a memento of a bygone past: they aim to be a lively cultural and social hub, a socially aware, relevant and responsive platform facilitating discourses around mental health's past, present and future. They aim to be a 'museum-laboratory'.[18] Whereas asylum museums are mainly about asylum staff and life, mind museums pursue a genuine attempt to open up their narrative and stories, take in different voices and promote individual reflection and engagement with the past and the present of mental health care. The relationship they have with the heritage they conserve and exhibit is not nostalgic or celebratory, nor overtly evolutionistic as it often is in asylum museums, but proactive and inquiring, aimed as it is at exploring the potential for this heritage to act as a door opener and to unlock new ways to talk about mental health today. Such vision, ambition and mission inform mind museums' work, with consequences on their collecting strategies, their display practices and exhibition design which are chiefly intended to retrieve previously excluded, overlooked and marginalised voices, stimulate reflections and bring diverse audiences together through the heritage of mental health.

Firstly, this is evident in their collecting strategies. Virtually all mind museums, within the limits of their own financial capacities, are engaged in active collecting through loans, encouraging donations, commissioning, acquisitions and as part of their outreach projects. Collecting is done with a primary focus on the most recent past and contemporary psychiatry and mental health stories. The overarching objective is to broaden their collections notably by including different and previously underrepresented voices, mainly those of people with lived experiences, including psychiatric survivors, service users and their families. Secondly, their more expansive mission is also reflected in the number, type and range of activities promoted by mind museums. Many of these activities are aimed at reaching out and actively engaging with a broad range of stakeholders and participants, notably including people with lived experiences and service users but also young adults and the general public at large. The span of activities promoted is quite broad and, as might be expected, varies in type and scale from institution to institution, according to their budget and specific focus. They generally involve guided and facilitated tours and educational programmes targeted at secondary school pupils (offered by virtually all such museums). They often also include temporary exhibitions and may extend to include artistic residencies and art projects, performances, music and theatre pieces and cultural festivals. These activities tap into the museum's collections and archives and often involve the active contribution of 'experts by experience', namely people who have recent personal experience of or caring for someone who has mental health problems and/or uses mental health social care services.

Examples abound. The *Museo Laboratorio della Mente* in Rome stands out for the number, variety and quality of the exhibitions, outreach, community and educational projects it promotes. From 2013 to 2018, it has promoted and run jointly with other cultural associations, NGOs, research centres and artists over ten major projects, including art projects, installations, travelling exhibitions, seminars and conferences (Fusco et al. 2019). Among these is the exhibition *Portatori di Storie* [*Bearers of Stories*], which opened in 2011 (Museo Laboratorio della Mente and Studio Azzurro 2019: 46–63). Drawing on a two-year project run by the museum in collaboration with the regional department of mental health, *Portatori di Storie* collects and displays the stories of 50 participants who are mental health workers, service users and their families. The exhibition has been designed by Studio Azzuro and is temporarily set up in the old hospital's library with the plan to move it within the main museum venue in pavilion No.6 of the former Santa Maria della Pietà psychiatric hospital, as part of its ongoing renewal. Like the museum's main exhibition, *Portatori di Storie* is based on a highly interactive interface, and it is a very immersive and emotional installation. Upon entering the old library room, the visitor find themselves among other people: they are the research participants' holograms projected on a screen, walking among the library's shelves. With a touch of the hand, the visitor can stop one of these persons who introduces themselves. Keeping the hand-contact, the visitor and this person can walk together into an adjacent smaller room; once there, the 'messenger' shares their story of lived experience and the visitor listens. The idea behind the installation is to perform an 'encounter' that, as any true encounter, changes and sometimes challenges those who experience it. The visitor may discover that who they thought was a nurse is actually a service user or a family member or the other way around; the visitor will learn about their personal struggles with mental health, its care and treatment, their success and failures. Some might feel upset, others relieved in hearing stories that resonate with their own experiences and feelings. Some may learn something they did not know or discover a different perspective on something they thought they knew. The exhibition is the incarnation of the museum's aim to be a 'laboratory', a place where knowledge is co-produced, dismantled and re-assembled, to raise questions and, using Martelli's words, to 'offer a space for reflection and possibly even dissent'.[19]

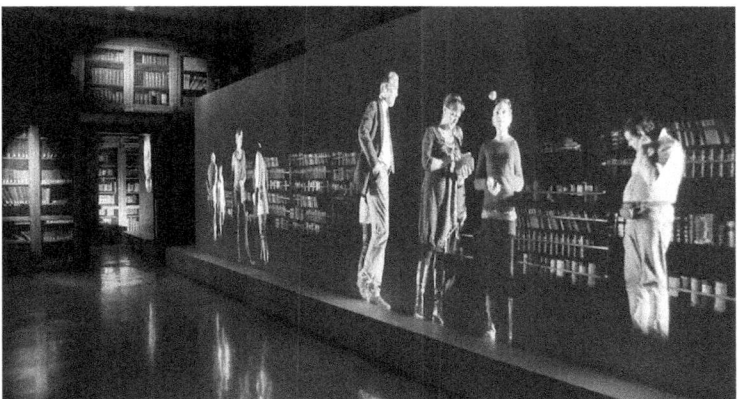

Image 2.10 Museo Laboratorio della Mente, Rome. Exhibition *Portatori di Storie*.

Exhibiting madness

As the exhibition *Portatori di Storie* ably illustrates, another key difference between asylum museums and mind museums aims can be observed in their exhibition design and display strategies. Whilst the exhibitions of the majority of asylum museums are somehow amateurish and often even self-produced, in mind museums their design is a key element in the overall museum project, and it often involves the contribution and the collaboration of professional designers and museum curators. Although the design of mind museums' exhibitions is not readily characterised by any particularly recurrent visual or curatorial strategy, it is possible to identify some recurrent features. We shall start by noting how, in the majority of mind museums, the display is structured in a linear narrative path and organised according to a thematic diachronic ordering by juxtaposing a selection of historical and contemporary objects from the museum collections. A similar tendency to move from chronological display logic, toward a diachronic thematic one, can be observed in other museums that have been currently undergoing a rethinking of their mission and strategies, such as, for example, city museums (Lanz 2012). In these museums, this approach allows to open up the museum's narrative to more contemporary urban issues connecting them with the city history – for example introducing displays and exhibitions focusing on migration and diversity and foster reflections about belonging and place identity (Lanz 2014). In mind museums such an approach is deployed to spotlight specific approaches to mental health treatment and care and to invite the visitor to look at them in perspective, connecting the past and present. Furthermore the different thematic highlights structuring each mind museum exhibition can be traced back to the museum's more or less patently declared position about contemporary mental health politics.

Another recurrent characterising trait in mind museums' exhibition is the abundant presence of a great number of historical textual resources; excerpts from former patients' medical records, letters, photos and other personal documents, in particular. This, in part, depends on the very nature of mind museums' historical collections, which often include a large amount of textual and archival materials. Furthermore, in many cases, mind museums' collections have been recently enlarged to incorporate oral history archives and other kinds of contemporary documents and resources that add to the 'less material' and personal bank of mind museums' collections. Nathan Flis and David Wright suggest that most recent mental health memorialisation practices, such as those at work in mind museums, borrow 'motifs ... from memorialisation of the Holocaust, the First World War, and American slavery [...] adapted to the political aspirations of "psychiatry survivors" organisations' (2011: 102). The authors do not expound much further on this remark in their paper; however, it can be argued that they are most probably referring to such extensive use in mind museums exhibitions of personal stories and direct witnesses. Whilst this observation is true in principle, such a turn to personal stories and memories can be seen more broadly in many contemporary museums, rather than being a specific feature of mind museums. It is particularly evident in exhibitions at museums, memorials and commemoration sites that deal with difficult, controversial and potentially contentious pasts and stories and wicked social problems. It is the case of Holocaust memorials, war museums, slavery museums, migration museums and sites of conscience more broadly, and crucially of mind museums too. Additionally it must be noted that the importance accorded to these documents and the key role entrusted to the display of these stories and resources in mind museums' exhibitions is also a consequence of their attempt to go beyond the mere display of asylum memorabilia and to achieve a all-rounded exploration of the heritage of mental health they conserve and exhibit also by reweaving the material culture, institutional histories and practices of the asylum with the micro-stories, personal lives and often-underrepresented voices of patients.

Above all, the exhibition and display strategies of mind museums are strongly linked to a foundational critical reflection on the past and contemporary politics of mental health that underpins and informs the overall museum project including its design. This position may vary, sometimes remarkably, from museum to museum – primarily because each institution is shaped by its specific national context, policies and politics of psychiatric care and assistance – and it may not be immediately readable within their display. Nevertheless, each mind museum's display is effectively conceived and designed to be a 'sophisticated form of political,

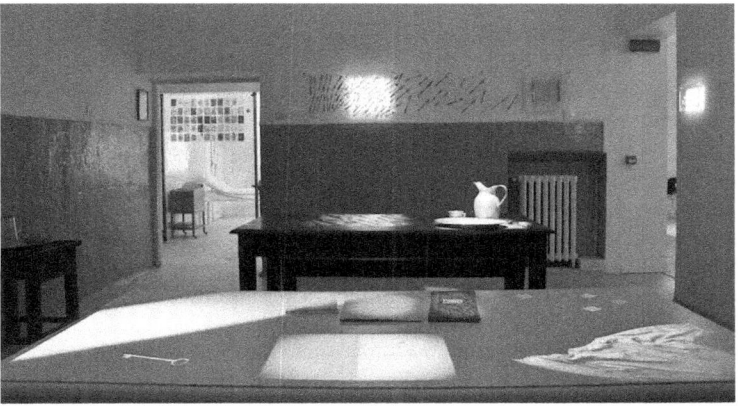

Image 2.11 Museo Laboratorio della Mente, Rome.
Display titled 'Storie' [stories] within the exhibition section *L'istituzione chiusa* ['The Closed Institution'].

public production of propositional knowledge intended to influence audiences and to create durable social effects' (Whitehead 2016b: 2). These 'effects' are geared towards promoting awareness, debate and reflections about the past and present of mental health, ultimately contributing to the dismantling of stigma and prejudices surrounding mental health today. The examples discussed below, based on a critical display analysis (Moser 2010; Lindauer 2006) of two mind museums' exhibitions, aim to illustrate and discuss this key point, as well as identify possible directions for future developments.

Virtually the whole exhibition at the *Museo Laboratorio della Mente* in Rome is made of stories and witnesses and revolves around visitors' interactions with them. In the museum's main exhibition, the last room of the section, *L'istituzione chiusa* ['The Closed Institution'], which is titled 'Storie' [stories], re-creates the former asylum canteen. A few original objects – a jug, a dish, a tray and a cup – are set on an old table of the original refectory. Next to it there is another table, displaying a replica of a patient's clinical case log, a book with asylum regulations and the nurses' duties and shifts register. A visitor can activate each object by touching it; namely, they can access a record of stories and documents related to the master topic associated with that object, i.e. respectively: asylum treatments, asylum rules and asylum daily life. Visitors can thus select and listen to different stories – in the form of audio recording and projections realised with the support of professional actors – from both asylum staff and patients.

Such resources are particularly difficult to exhibit because of their immaterial or bi-dimensional nature, and their display often requires an elaborate exhibition design solution for their *mise-en-scène*. Through different exhibitionary and scenographic strategies, such staging aims at providing them with the visual strength they lack while at the same time fully exploiting and empowering their significance, emotional depth and empathetic potential often aimed at visitors' active affective, intellectual and physical interactions. In some cases, as happens more widely in museums dealing with difficult heritage, this is done by resorting to new digital and emerging technologies (Stylianou-Lambert et al. 2022). In many cases, it involves a juxtaposition of these textual and more immaterial resources, personal stories and witnesses with other more visually compelling and materially tangible collection items and the material culture of the asylum, notably including some 'iconic objects'. These are objects from the museum's collection that are characterised by a strong visual impact and immediate connection with mental health and the asylum. Beyond the historic or artistic value iconic objects may have, their place and role in mind museums' display lies in the meanings they embody, the memories they evoke and in their scenographical impact. They are, we may say, the opposite of memorabilia, meaning 'objects valued for their original association with the period itself rather than for their informational and educational value' (Macdonald 2005: 222), not in their nature but in the way they are understood and used. Some iconic objects of mind museums' exhibitions, in fact, are ubiquitous in asylum museums, too; most notably, straitjackets and medical restraints tools, padded cells and containment beds and ECT machines. What distinguishes their display in mind museums compared to asylum museums is the conscious and genuine attempt to shy away from voyeuristic drifts, to avoid poignancy that may lead to pity, and rather to capitalise on their power to spur emphatic reaction in visitors as a starting point to prompt personal reflections around past and contemporary ideas and stereotypes about mental health care.

The current exhibition of the *Bethlem Museum of the Mind* offers perfect examples of all three exhibition design features mentioned above: thematic diachronic ordering; the use of textual resources, micro-stories and personal witnesses; and the role of iconic objects. I visited the museum in July 2021, soon after it had reopened after the pandemic. As already mentioned, the exhibition is organised into three main thematic sections: 'Labelling and Diagnosis', 'Freedom and Constraint' and 'Heal or Harm'. The main display of the 'Labelling and Diagnosis' section features a selection of photographic portraits realised by Brian Moody and accompanied by original written personal narratives collected by Marina Cantacuzino for the 2002 travelling exhibition *1 in 4*[20] alongside other historical prints, drawing, physiognomic studies and portraits from the Bethlem asylum's Victorian photos archive. Some of them are framed and hung on the walls; others are displayed in the drawers of an archive-like file case that can be opened and browsed by the visitor. Other objects on display include an historical admission register of the asylum, where a diagnosis was noted for each patient admitted at the hospital, contemporary service users' artworks with annotation on how these are often used to assess patients' mental health status and a desktop station providing access to the online encyclopaedia of mental illness. The display's key intent is challenging stereotypes, biases and mistakes within and beyond the medical practices about how madness 'looks'; it invites the visitor to begin reflecting on the subtle and questionable boundary between a diagnosis and a label and on the ethics of patients' classification. Given that a medical diagnosis in the United Kingdom may determine a person's possibility to choose whether they do or do not want to be treated and even their freedom to accept or decline hospital admission, I found these questions are extremely rich with implications.

The section 'Labelling and Diagnosis' ends at the threshold of the new museum extension. This is a small-sized space creating a sort of buffer area, in between the section on 'Labelling and Diagnosis' and the one focusing on 'Freedom and Constraints'. Walking through a small door carved out of the historical building's thick wall, I enter a small, almost empty white and naturally lit space. The space feels almost wall-less, with a large floor-to-ceiling window. This is the only outward-looking window in the whole exhibition space; it looks out over the hospital park, creating a strong visual connection between the museum interior spaces and the hospital site. Standing in front of this large window, I felt projected outwards where the hospital parkland extends as far as the eye can see with open grass fields, beautiful flower beds and trees, fenced gardens looked after by service users and newly built residential units that are, to me, easily distinguishable from other non-residential pavilions for their surrounding iron wireframe or wood made high fence walls (about freedom and constraint).

The space features only one exhibit: a 20th-century padded cell, one of the master iconic objects in exhibitions and displays about asylums. However, I only noticed this a few moments after I had entered the space because the padded panels and the door of the isolation room are mounted on the wall beyond the visitor's shoulders. The information panel includes an excerpt from a 1970 account of a patient about her experience of detention in a padded cell; the text talks about the practice of isolating patients in the past and the present and how 'the freedom of the countryside is at the other end of the scale from the experience of confinement in a padded cell' (from the 'In and Out' panel, Bethlem Museum of the Mind, July 2021). Again, more questions arose in my mind: Is there freedom in confinement? Knowing that involuntary hospitalisation and treatment are today allowed in the United Kingdom under the national mental health act, does this remote and pleasant countryside location really represent the opposite of a padded cell? Isn't it just another and more subtle form of isolation?

'The balance between freedom and constraint has always been contested in mental healthcare, and has repeatedly challenged medical practice and the law' – I read in the introductory panel of the following section, 'Freedom and Constraints'. This section is quite visually and intellectually compelling. A large frame-less glass case with a contemporary style is filled with tens of historical glass bottles and lit with coloured led lights intermittently switching from red – an intense and exciting colour that may evoke a state of uproar but also fear – to green – a colour instead broadly associated with calm and nature. In front of it there is a 19th-century straitjacket: like the padded cell, this is another recurrent iconic object of mental health exhibitions (Coleborne 2001). The straitjacket is displayed in another frameless glass case; next to it there is a mirror reflecting several 18th-century restraint devices hung on the back side of a white wall, meaning they cannot be seen in any way other than through the mirror. The accompanying label and the information panel remark and expand on how the straitjacket was in fact introduced as part of non-restraint approaches. The question asked aloud here is whether contemporary psychiatric practices and devices such as physical handling, compulsory treatment orders, drug treatments, electronic tagging and CCTV monitoring in psychiatric hospitals wards are themselves nothing but other forms of freedom limitations and controls, just like the straitjacket. Where is the line between consideration for patient care and safety, on the one hand, and the denial of freedom and control on the other?

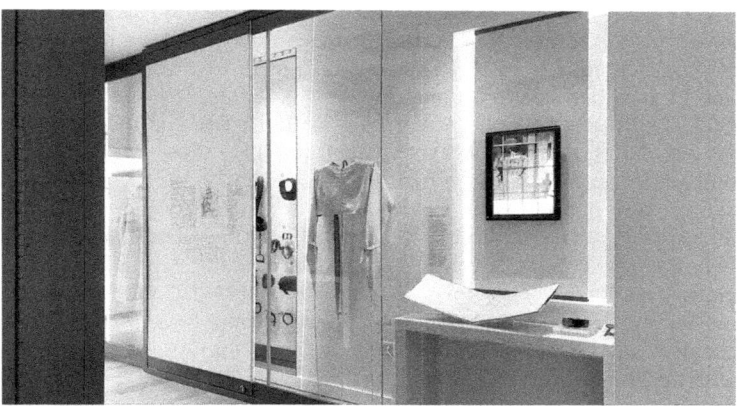

Image 2.12 Bethlem Museum of the Mind. Straitjacket display in the section 'Freedom and Constraints'.
Photo by Francesca Lanz, July 2021.

These questions are piling up and resonating with one another in my mind, when I finally enter the final section, 'Heal or Harm'. Here, I encounter another ever-present iconic object, the ECT machine. ECT (electroconvulsive therapy) was originally developed in 1937 by the Italian psychiatric and neurologist Ugo Cerletti with Lucio Bini for the treatment of schizophrenic patients. It is still in use today as a medical treatment, especially offered to people suffering from severe, drug-resistant and life-threatening depressive syndromes (Pancheri and Caredda 1999). While published scientific studies, supported also by *American Psychiatric Association* and the *Royal College of Psychiatrists*, show improvements in patients' conditions for up to about 75–80% of patients, the long-term benefits of ECT treatment are an open matter of discussion. Major concerns are possible side effects, including permanent memory losses, and some suggest that ECT may worsen patients' life quality in the long run. For these reasons, the advantages and disadvantages of ECT are currently under study and a matter of debate and evaluation within the scientific community. However, debate on the use of ECT in contemporary psychiatric treatment involves more than medical science and ethics, but also personal opinions, influenced by lived experiences as much as by collective imaginary, as well as by political and ideological positions. As such, the debate extends far beyond the medical sphere (e.g. the Church of Scientology has always campaigned strongly against psychiatric treatments, the use of ECT in particular).

The ECT mobilises memories from a not-so-remote past, when first attempts in the use of electroconvulsive procedures for therapeutic purposes were extremely tentative and prone to errors but also to unethical experimentation on unwilling patients. Not infrequently, ECT was misused as one of the possible fall-back solutions, extreme yet handy, in overcrowded wards to tranquilise those who were too difficult to manage and as a form of punishment to restore power and control (Goffmann 1961). For those with lived experience of asylum internment, who underwent ECT therapy during their stay, and for their relatives, the sole term 'electroshock' recalls painful and traumatic experiences. The work of Alda Merini (1931–2009), an Italian writer and poet nominated in 1996 for the Nobel Prize in Literature, provides a vivid account of this. Her writings and poems are infused with her lived experience, which was marked by institutionalisation in several different Italian asylums at the end of the 1960s, in particular, the Paolo Pini mental hospital in Milan, during which she underwent involuntary treatments, including ECT. In most people's imaginations, the ECT is straightforwardly associated with the asylum, broadly imagined as an uncaring and dehumanised place of social isolation, custody and harm. It triggers dreadful images, such as those from the well-known 1975 movie by Miloš Forman, *One Flew on the Cuckoo's Nest*, where ECT was used for punitive purposes on a perfectly sane McMurphy (played by Jack Nicholson) by cold and detached doctors and nurses. It does not require a great imaginative leap from here to reviving nightmarish images of Dr. Frankestein–like experimentation, torture and even the electric chair. During my fieldwork in former asylums' historical archives, more than once I found myself puzzled and upset by browsing treatment logs and patients' medical records and skimming line after line of ECT treatments repeatedly administered to the same person for several days in a row, with no other annotation than date and voltage details, in some cases simply complemented by a few cursory notes on the patient clinical response to the treatment. Many times, I could not prevent my mind from drifting in eerie speculations. Almost every mind museum includes an ECT machine in its display.

The debate around the use of ECT treatment is extremely emblematic of how mental health care has always been an area of medical study and practice particularly rich in uncertainties, unknowns and controversies characterised by an uncommon and deep intertwinement between science and medical debate, politics, public opinion and personal experience. It makes it evident how, when talking about madness, it is extremely difficult to draw a line between medical science, evidence and our own imagination and fears. At the *Bethlem Museum of the Mind*, in the exhibition section titled 'Heal and Harm', two electrotherapy machines and associated equipment from the mid-20th century are displayed beyond a glass window together with a two-episode documentary on the use of ECT realised by Jim Reed for the BBC Newsnight and first broadcast on BBC2 on July 2013.[21] A museum volunteer, during an informal conversation with me, mentioned the very strong and emotional reaction of a visitor to this display for she had been given shock therapy in the past. Duncan Dudley, in his dissertation on visitor emotional reaction to exhibitions on mental health, remarks on how this 'video was noted by a number of visitors as being particularly unexpected and upsetting' (2018). I found this display very informative and thought-provoking. Throughout the exhibition, but foremost in this display, is an invitation to the visitor to reflect on the conflict between care and control, care and abuse, and whether and at which extent in mental health care medical considerations should or not prevail over individual freedom and the individual's right to choose.

At the end of my long and very emotionally and intellectually dense visit to the small *Bethlem Museum of the Mind*, I had a walk in the surrounding park. The museum is, after all, located in the premises not of a former asylum but of a still-functioning psychiatric hospital and I wanted to understand, experience, and read the museum within its context, for the key questions of my study revolved in fact around mind museums' nature as place-based and site-specific cultural institutions. For asylum museums, their location within the premises of a former asylum location is often chosen (better say given) mainly in continuity with their formation and for practical and pragmatic reasons: it is therefore taken for granted and rarely given critical consideration. As noted earlier, in asylum museums, the building hosting the museum is not usually the object of any significant intervention other than those most basically needed to make it immediately accessible and usable (probably also due to the lack of resources) and the overall historical context where the museum is located, is not considered for its potential contribution to the museum narrative; even less, it is utilised in any significant way as a platform for the museum work or integrated in any way into its display and design. Paradoxically, in asylum museums former asylum architectural spaces are often 'recreated' in their exhibitions through historical reconstructions of specific rooms or dioramas, while very little attention is focused instead to the spaces occupied by the museums itself, which are in effect themselves 'real' places of the asylum.

This is very evident, for example, at the *Glenside Hospital Museum* described earlier. However, also at the *Bethlem Museum of the Mind,* the relationship between the museum and the site is quite ambiguous: apart from some references to the importance of the park as public space used and appreciated by the whole Beckenham community, the actual place out there, namely a still working psychiatric hospital, tends to disappear in the museum display. The sole exception is the small extension room, but whether this was intentionally designed this way to compel the kind of reaction and thoughts I had there remains to be clarified. The *Museo Laboratorio della Mente* once more offers a good example. In 2008, when the museum was being renovated to turn it from an exhibition on the history of the asylum to a mind museum, considerable attention and funds were invested in the design of the new exhibition, minimum interventions were done on the built fabric of the former asylum pavilion housing it. Interior spaces were painted white, very few original features were left in place and nothing helps the visitor to understand what the pavilion was and how it appeared. Outward-looking windows are blinded, not least because the exhibition heavily relies on projections and therefore requires dark spaces. Because of that, the very immersive nature of the exhibition and the overall neutral and anonymous interior spaces where it is set up, the visitor can easily forget that they are in the pavilion of a former asylum. Most recently however, the *Museo Laboratorio della Mente* has been increasingly and significantly investing in strengthening the relationship between the museum and its context, for example by creating site-specific installations and promoting site-specific projects. The ongoing renovation project also will focus more on the museum building's materiality and traces. Overall, compared to asylum museums, mind museums engage with their site more reflexively, looking at it as a key component of their identity and work. Former asylum sites, for their nature as palimpsests, hold the potential to act as power places of awareness; the place could greatly support mind museums in their mission, determining not only what they are, but also, crucially, what do they do or may do and with which effects. However, at the moment, the relationship between mind museums and their site as well as their nature as place-based institutions seem to be more of potential aspects of what these museums are and do rather than characterising and consolidated features.

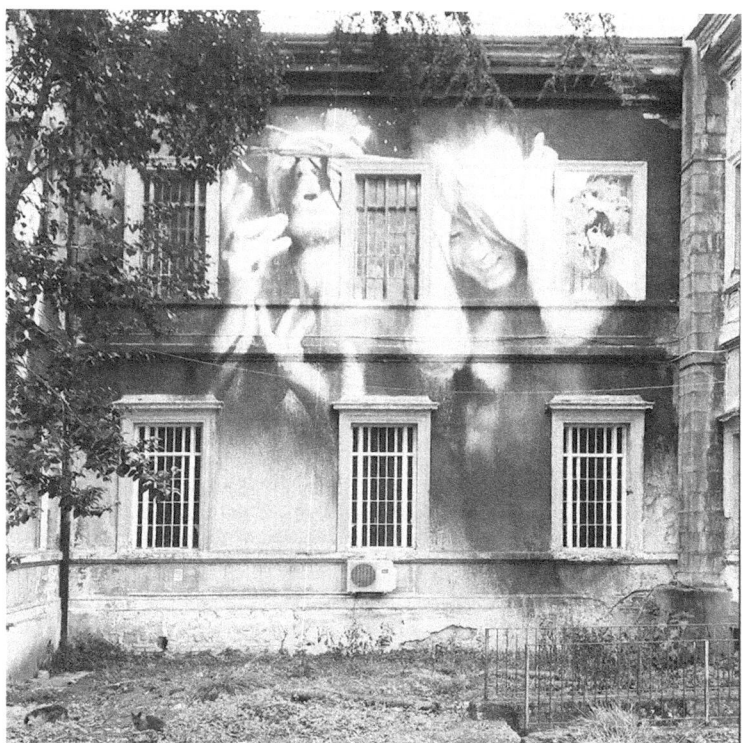

Image 2.13 Pavilion no. 6 of the former psychiatric hospital Santa Maria della Pietà, Roma.
Site-specific murales *Le cose che non si vedono* [Things that Are Not Seen], by Luis Gomez de Teran realised for *Museo Laboratorio della Mente*. Foto di Francesca Lanz, dicembre 2019.

Notes

1 I here adopt Whitehead's definition of display as a 'sophisticated form of representation and communication that aims to present particular narratives or organizations of knowledge, or to create sensory environments and affective spaces that invite or impel visitors to respond in a certain way' (2016a: 2; 2016b) and as a 'political, public production of propositional knowledge intended to influence audiences and to create durable social effects' (2016b: 2).
2 Mason et al. compare displays to other forms of written histories and highlight how their distinctive aspect is being in architectural space and they are 'physical, spatial, aural, sometimes emotional and affecting, always embodied' (2018b: 56).
3 See also Introduction.

4 Psychiatric photography was introduced at the San Lazzaro asylum by superintendent doctor Augusto Tamburni, who managed the asylum from 1877 to 1907 and introduced a number of innovations, including the systematic use of clinical logs and the opening of the first vocational training course for nurses.

5 In Italy, the preservation and conservation of former asylums' archives – former patients' casebooks in particular – their study and critical interpretation have fostered the development of several research projects of different scales and has been a key driving factor in the birth of asylum and mind museums in the country. In 1999, the research programme *Carte da Legare* [Binding Cards] has been initiated by the Italian Ministry for Cultural Heritage and Activities and Tourism (MIBACT) in collaboration with the Italian National Archive Network, with the overarching objective to promote the study, preservation and valorisation of the archival and documental heritage of mental health. *Carte da Legare* promoted the first comprehensive census of all the Italian former asylums' archives. It has been an umbrella project for several smaller-scale and site specifics projects aimed at the inventory and digitalisation of asylum patients' clinical logs conserved in former Italian asylums' archives which have been carried out by universities and research centres in collaboration with scientific libraries, local health units (ASL – *Aziende Sanitarie Locali*) and the museums that today are entrusted for the conservation and preservation of former asylum archives and collections. Data collected and catalogued can be consulted online for research purposes via the digital portal *Carte da Legare* (*Carte da Legare* n.d.). A similar project was *Gli Spazi della Follia* [The Spaces of Madness], also connected with MIBACT and the national Italian Archives Network, an open access database of historical documents pertaining to 19th-century asylums' historical architectural complexes and reporting on their conservation status. The project drew on the findings of a national research project funded in 2018 by the Italian Ministry of Research and University (MIUR) that expanded and updated previous research carried out from 1996 to 1998 by the *Fondazione Benetton Studi e Ricerche* (Ajroldi et al. 2013; Crippa and Galliani 2013; Luciani 1999; *Gli Spazi della Follia* n.d.). Today, in Italy, there are several cultural associations of different kinds, including five museums that run activities, organise exhibitions and promote research, study and communication programme revolving around the heritage of mental health and with the aim of conserving, studying and valorising former historical asylums, their archives and collections. Several of them recently formed a nationwide network called *Mente in Rete* [Mind on the Net] (*Mente in Rete* n.d.). Established in 2018 and quickly growing in the number of its associate members, the network is meant to function as a platform to spur and facilitate debate and sharing among different institutions working with the heritage of mental health.

6 Art workshop and art therapy had been always encouraged in asylums for both leisure and therapeutic purposes, especially during the 20th century. Not only some psychiatrists initiated collecting art brute done by asylum inmates within and in some case even beyond their own institution, but also some private collectors became interested in this art, assembling sometimes relatively large collections.

7 In 2007, Rolf Brüggemann and Gisela Schmid-Krebs, who are respectively a psychologist and therapist at the Christophsbad psychosomatic hospital, both working at *MuSeele,* the museum of the history of psychiatry in Goppingen (Germany), published a book that reports on their personal visits to several psychiatry museums across Europe. The book overall includes over 60 asylum

and mental health museums, plus other examples of museums and cultural centres that they name as 'memorials of Ns-Euthanasia'; museums of 'the art of different kind' (i.e. museums with collection of art brute or outsider art); and 'elsewhere' (i.e. other museums they visited and that incorporated displays on the history of psychiatry and mental health) (Brüggemann and Schmid-Krebs 2007). Bronwyn Labrum (2011), in her essay on the exhibition of cloth and the representation of madness in museum displays, describes two asylum museums in Australia with remarkable similarities with other European asylum and mental health museums I could visit as part of my research.

8 The Former Glenside Hospital; today, it is the Glenside Campus of the University of West of England (UWE) hosting the faculty of Health and Applied Sciences since 1996.

9 In 1997, the museum's collection has further enlarged with the objects donated by staff members of the nearby Stoke Park Hospitals for Learning Disabilities which was about to close.

10 When visiting, it is not uncommon to do that with the accompaniment of the original organ played by the same former asylum staff member who played it back in time.

11 As emerged from the three visitors' books consulted during fieldwork and the data of a survey-based visitors study campaign run by the museum in 2019 involving over 400 participants. Courtesy of GHM.

12 Many research participants in my study draw a direct connection between asylums and concentration camps and torture.

13 The Santa Maria della Pietà asylum was designed according to the dictates of the moral approach by the architect Edgardo Negri. It occupied an area of about 150 hectares comprising 42 buildings, including services, pavilions, and a farm that were disposed in the landscape following its natural hill-shaped form and as a unified architectural project based on a village layout. The Santa Maria della Pietà asylum soon became a reference design model for other asylums in the country.

14 The acrylic wall features a full-scale reproduction of a fragment of NOF4 graffiti realised on the wall of the *Ferri* pavilion in the Volterra asylum (Studio Azzurro realised the film *L'osservatorio nucleare del sig Nanof* inspired to Nannetti's work in 1984, which was an inspiration for the design of the *Museo Laboratorio della Mente*'s exhibition.

15 Due to run until 31 December 2023.

16 Data extracted from Duncan Dudley's unpublished PhD dissertation (Dudley 2018) and GHM visitor survey run in 2019, courtesy of the GHM museum.

17 As mentioned in the preceding chapter, this is the case of the *Museo Laboratorio della Mente* in Roma, founded in 2000 by its current director, Dr Pompeo Martelli, a therapist who formerly worked at the mental hospital Santa Maria della Pieta in Rome (Italy) or the *Museo di Arte Paolo Pini – MAPP* in Milan, born in 1993 from a project by Teresa Melorio and Enza Baccei, respectively, a psychiatrist and psychologist working at the former Paolo Pini asylum in the years of its dismissal. Similarly, outside of Italy, the *Dr Guislain Museum* in Gent was created in the 1980s by Dr René Stockman, general director of the Dr. Guislain Psychiatric Centre at the time the museum was established.

18 Pompeo Martelli, when asked about what the *Museo Laboratorio della Mente* is, defined it as a 'museum' and a 'laboratory'. Both terms are included in the name given to the museum in 2008, because they, in combination, reflect its ambition to be an authoritative and trustworthy yet continuously changing

and evolving institution: to 'offer a space for reflection and possibly even dissent' (interview with Pompeo Martelli 22/11/2021). Similarly, Teresa Melorio told me that the decision to call the *MAPP* a 'museum', although the activities it promotes stretch far beyond those traditionally at the core of a museum institution, is because they recognise a strong transformative power to contemporary museums' work and their nature as safe spaces for difficult conversations, which they sought for the *MAPP* as well (interview with Teresa, 20/04/2022).

19 From the interview with Pompeo Martelli 22/11/2021.
20 Organised in 2002 as part of a mental health campaign run by the Department of Health.
21 https://www.bbc.co.uk/news/av/health-23453426 [Last Accessed, July 2022].

3   Re-mind museums

Despite being the smallest among the contemporary European mind museums discussed so far, and although its identity is still situated somewhere between that of an asylum museum and a mind museum, the *Museo di Storia della Psichiatria* (Museum of the History of Psychiatry) in Reggio Emilia, Italy, has been selected as a key example. This choice is made because it most clearly links its historical collection with its site and intentionally leverages such heritage as a resource for promoting knowledge and awareness about mental health care in the past and present. This final chapter revolves around the discussion of this single case study, drawing on extensive fieldwork carried out at the museum to address some of the key questions posed in this book regarding the relationship existing at mind museums between site materiality, associated memories, and the overall museum project, and to delve into their combined role in determining visitors' museum experience and its effects.

Methodological note

Fieldwork for my study was planned to start in early spring 2020; It notably included visitor studies campaing in selected museums across Europe, which were intended to provide me with insights into how people react to a highly layered, memory-laden and evocative spatial context such as the one characterising mind museums, and how they make sense out of it. To that aim, this aspect of the study hinged on a set of on-site and face-to-face qualitative interviews incorporating 'tripartite' model of pre- and post-visit interviews using the 'thinking aloud' method (Hooper-Greenhill and Moussouri 2001); observations of visitors' in-gallery emotional behaviours; and 'walkthrough' methods, consisting in first-person perspective video recordings of visits using a head-mounted camera, with video data analysis complemented by follow-up interview (Allen et al. 2014; Mason et al. 2018b; Pink 2015; Pink et al. 2017). However, the COVID-19 outbreak, and the associated restrictions aimed at limiting the spread of the virus, made it impossible

DOI: 10.4324/9781003258971-4

to carry out fieldwork as planned. At first, I paused site visits and considered implementing a contingency plan to carry out visitor studies relying on methods conceived to achieve similar ends. However, I soon realised that the changed context required not just an adjustment in timing and methods for my fieldwork and visitor studies, but a profound rethinking of their structure and ultimate purpose. The original methods had been chosen for their potential to spur and record the participants' immediate responses to the museum's display and spatial context. They would have supported me in assessing the role of the museum's display and spatial context in provoking emotional reactions in visitors and fostering heritage-emotion-based reflections on mental health issues. With the museum closed indefinitely and new visit protocols in place, it was unlikely that my interviews could draw on participants' fresh, physical experiences of the museum and their affective reactions to the visit.

I eventually decided to redesign my fieldwork as a multi-tasked exploration chiefly focused on one case study. It involved literature and archival research,[1] solo visits, and visitor observations at a distance, remote interviews with experts via email and using on-line videoconferencing platforms, and two campaigns of remote and in-person visitor studies. Most importantly I decided to carry out the main campaign of visitor studies remotely, shifting its focus from exploring how people react to museum displays and spatial contexts during the visit, to their recollections of that experience: How do visitors make sense of their visit *time after it*? What bodies, interfaces, technologies and devices are active within the acts of remembering? Which kinds of emotions and reflections have been sustained in people's memories after the visit? Taking this approach presented me with new methodological challenges. It required me to think about methods that could help me capturing and exploring non-cognitive, emotive and embodied understandings associated with a visit experience – a challenge amplified by the fact that the visitor studies would now happen at a distance, both in time and space. All that involved looking for alternative ways to create the condition for these memories to arise, and the essential intimacy and feeling of trustfulness needed to address such questions, without relying on the physical proximity of either the research participants and the researchers or the site itself.

'If we want to think about the messiness of reality at all then we're going to have to teach ourselves to think, to practice, to relate, and to know in new ways' said John Law (2004: 2). In the introduction of his book, *After Methods*, Law invites us to embrace blindness, uncertainty, imprecision and dead-ends not as obstacles but for what they can offer to our research. An opportunity that, by slowing our work, might impede us from learning about certain things but may also allow us to learn about a 'wider range of realities'. The point that he makes is that the world is all but homogeneous, steady or secure and, given that the methods we use produce the realities into which they enquire, methods seeking for certainty may distort into clarity the world they aim to describe. What Law suggests is that we should also look for research methods that are capable of studying the indefinite and irregular. To do so, he says, we shall engage with these realities, renouncing our eagerness to fix them, but rather exploring these realities by adopting unusual methods, 'different forms of knowing' and a different, 'broader or more generous sense of method'. This is how he introduces and then further articulates his idea of 'method assemblage': an 'enactment of relations', and 'a combination of reality detector and reality amplifier'. Law's idea resonated in meaningful and inspiring ways with my research struggles, and it shed a different light on my approach to visitor studies. It prompted me to rethink and reconsider the kind of methods I wanted to deploy and how I could adapt them productively and creatively to the new context. Seeking 'different forms of knowing' and a more 'generous sense of methods', I redesigned my visitor studies as remote, unstructured narratives and visual, emotionally elicited interviews.

Interview were carried out with whomever had visited the museum at least once at any time and revolved around a few probing questions. These were characterised by flexibility and openness and aimed at probing participants about their reflective answers. As in narrative interviews, the participants were asked to narrate their experience for the researcher, shifting the way interview roles are usually conceptualised: from interviewer–interviewee into narrator–listener (Edwards & Holland, 2013; Kartch 2017). To fill the temporal and physical gap between the interview and the visit experience, the participant and me, us and the site, I resorted to photo and video elicitation. Harper points out, 'photo elicitation interview seems like not simply an interview process that elicits more information, but rather one that evokes a different kind of information' (Harper 2002: 13) and allows researchers and their participants to talk and learn about them differently.

Photo elicitation – explains Harper – 'is based on the simple idea of inserting a photograph into a research interview' (2002: 13) to prompt participants' responses (Banks and Zeitlyn 2015: 86–94; Harper 2002; Pink 2013: 92–102; Rose 2012: 297–327).[2] Photographs are recognised as means evoking deeper elements of human consciousness, sharpening and eliciting different kind of knowledge and memories and stimulating emotional statements, as well as enhancing the sensory dimension of the interview. Previous studies relying on photo elicitation techniques, moreover, demonstrate that photos can also help the interview flow more naturally and adaptively, as well as allowing the articulation (in verbal and non-verbal ways) thoughts and feeling that may otherwise remain silent, implicit or unseen, and prompt a discussion that adopts different registers, which are usually more emotional and affective. Furthermore, as photographs do not contain meanings in themselves, as Sarah Pink reminds us, in photo elicitation interviews, knowledge is not extracted from the image but 'constituted through the image' and co-created by the participant and the researcher and photographic meanings are 'renegotiated and remade' in the interview context as part of the process of creating knowledge (Pink 2013:99). This is why photo elicitation is considered a method that is very much a process, tapping into emotional and sensory knowledge dimensions, and that requires a core collaboration between the researchers and an empowerment of the participants more than other methods do. As such, it not only helped me in creating a feeling of intimacy with the research participants but also in gaining more and different insights on their visit experience, and to do that using 'different forms of knowing' (Law 2004), including knowing as 'embodiment', 'emotionality', as 'situated inquiry' and through 'techniques of deliberate imprecision' (Law 2004: 2–3) and as 'empathising' (Pink et al. 2017).

Photo elicitation methodologies also differ significantly in the way the data gathered from the interview are subsequently analysed by the researchers, although this is often done accounting for both the visual and the textual data and the relationship between the two, as well as the participants' interaction with and reaction to the images. Photo elicitation is an open and flexible methodology, as Shanti Sumartojo remarks, it is not only the how-to-do photo elicitation that can change but also, and more crucially, the actual rationale beyond the choice of deploying and adapting these techniques, which can evolve and develop from project to project and within the same project in response to evolving and emerging needs (Sumartojo 2019: 27). In this sense, as an ongoing process of making methods and developing analytical activities, photo elicitation offered me the 'broad and generous' methodology I was looking for. After three mock interviews and two pilots to test different interviewing methods, visitor studies at the *Museo di Storia della Psichiatria* eventually started in January 2021 and concluded in July 2021. The results of this study are presented in this final chapter.

The *Museo di Storia della Psichiatria* in Reggio Emilia: A case study

The *Museo di Storia della Psichiatria* is housed in the Lombroso pavilion within the former San Lazzaro mental asylum of Reggio Emilia, in the north of Italy (Ajroldi et al. 2013: 223–225; Grassi et al. 2013; Lanz 2020; Lanz and Montanari 2022; Tagliabue 2013). The history of the San Lazzaro is similar to those of many other asylums in Italy and abroad. It was established in the early 19th century on the eastern outskirts of the city of Reggio Emilia. Throughout the 19th century, it grew and became famous all over Italy and Europe. At the beginning of the 20th century, it was a sort of small, self-sufficient town, which included more than 20 buildings organised in a cottage plan, with about 2,000 patients hospitalised every year – for a period, one of these was the renowned Italian artist Antonio Ligabue (1899–1965). During the 20th century, the hospital started a slow but relentless decline: officially closed by law in 1978, the last patients were eventually dismissed in 1997. Even before its official closure, and definitively afterwards, no funding was invested in the asylum. This meant that only very basic maintenance was carried out on its aging structures; the complex thus quickly started to decay, and several pavilions were progressively dismissed for obsolescence and redundancy and abandoned. The Lombroso was one of these.

Originally named Casino Galloni, the pavilion dates back to 1892 and it was devoted to hosting 'calm chronic patients'. In 1911, after the *Legge Giolitti* in 1904 imposed the creation of specific forensic sections in psychiatric hospitals for the isolation of 'mad criminals', the Casino Galloni was converted for this purpose. It was enlarged by adding two lateral wings hosting the inmates' cells and named after the doctor Cesare

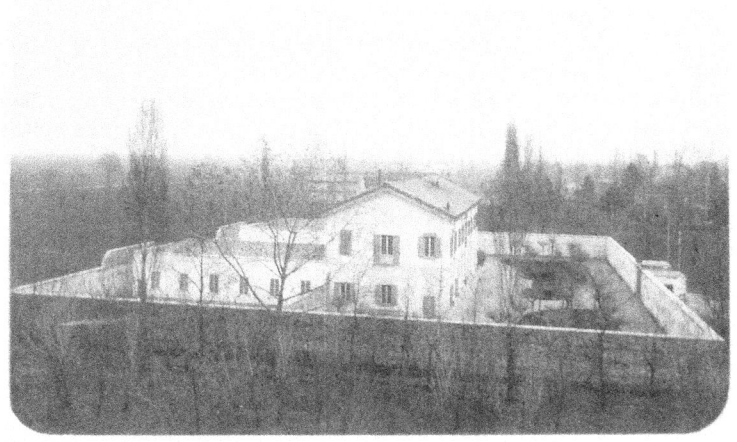

Image 3.1 San Lazzaro mental asylum, Reggio Emilia, Italy.
Photo of the Lombroso pavilion. Photo realised for the 1910 World Expo. Source: Archive of the former San Lazzaro psychiatric hospital, Scientific Library Carlo Livi, Reggio Emilia. Archive code: RESL0193. Available in the public domain.

Lombroso. Minor changes were made to the Lombroso throughout its life span and it was used until its abandonment in 1972 and the now-disused pavilion's containment wall was demolished in 1974. Already before the hospital's official closure, there was an idea to establish a museum at the former San Lazzaro asylum in the Lombroso pavilion. However, even though a call for project was launched in 1978 (Bergomi 1980), the museum was not realised, and the pavilion continued to decay, as did the whole site.

In 2009, an urban rehabilitation plan for the whole San Lazzaro estate — 296,792 sqm — was approved by the municipality. It involved major works to regenerate the area, converting it into a mixed-function urban public space, including public health service facilities hosted in the reused premised of former asylum pavilions, spaces for the city's public university, a public park and a museum of the history of the asylum, to be hosted in the former Lombroso pavilion. When the works for the rehabilitation and reuse of the former San Lazzaro complex started, the asylum was still resonating in the city's memory in many ways, despite the fact that it had been closed and abandoned for more than a decade. As discussed in the first chapters, the asylum had been an important element of the city's life and its development, even after its closure and abandonment, almost everyone in Reggio Emilia knew the San Lazzaro, from direct experience or hearsay. At the same time, whilst it was well known by almost all citizens, it was also a 'mysterious' and 'ghostly' place in the collective imaginary with 'stories' and 'legends' about the asylum circulating within the local communities.

The San Lazzaro was not a totally unknown place either to Giorgia Lombardini, the architect working at the technical office of the Reggio Emilia council in charge for the museum project, although she had never been there before 2006 when she carried out her first preliminary site survey. Before her inspection, she told me during our interview, many had advised her that due to the advanced status of decay of the Lombroso pavilion, 'there was nothing special there that could be valorised by any kind of restorative intervention'.[3] Therefore, most of her colleagues at the municipality technical office, when discussing the kind of intervention strategy to be adopted to convert the building into a museum, were quite keen on major alterations to the building fabric. However, after she visited the site, she saw it differently. 'Despite the manifest deterioration — she wrote in her report of the survey — the place emanates an atmosphere of rare uniqueness; at a closer look, one less superficial and more sensitive, beyond the stained surfaces and the ruining structures, the place allows to be half-seen extraordinary potentialities and a remarkable formal and aesthetic value' (Lombardini n.d.). This encounter with the place determined her design approach in museal conversion of the pavilion (Lanz 2020; Lanz and Montanari 2022).

The intervention on the Lombroso pavilion has been largely 'restorative' in its approach and techniques. Aimed as it was at 'maintaining intact the peculiar atmosphere of the place' (Lombardini n.d.), the intervention sought to conserve the spatial material features of the building fabric. The project adopted the guiding principle of 'integrating' what was missing not by replacing it, but rather by 'evoking the same aesthetic impression' (*ibid.*). It involved several accurate site surveys, including stratigraphic analysis campaigns and in-depth archival and historical research carried out with the support of Chiara Bombardieri — director of the *Biblioteca Scientifica Carlo Livi* and future chief curator of museum — who acted as scientific consultant for the whole project. Structural interventions on the building have been realised either adopting the same techniques and materials in the case of refurbishment, or with self-evident interventions in the case of new additions (such as the steel tie-rod structure aimed at reinforcing the floors and improve the seismic reaction or making new technical systems and wiring clearly distinguishable). Wall surfaces have been cleaned, scrubbing away squatters' graffiti and soot from interior fires. The more recent paint layers have been removed to reveal the original 19th-century mamorino wall plaster and the graffiti done by patients on the pavilion walls at different times using spoons and shoe soles, which have been professionally restored. Some of these graffiti include writings and others are more graphic; one of the larger is a mind map of the territory outside of Reggio Emilia, with annotations about places and villages — all named Busana, probably the patient's hometown.

Other architectural elements and details and furniture, such as the cell doors, windows and blinders and floor-mounted benches have been restored or philologically reconstructed. As part of the reuse intervention, the original containment wall that was demolished in 1974 has been also 'recreated': rebuilt on the same size and location of the former one, but with a wireframe structure in corten steel to evoke the former wall and serving as a support for temporary outdoor exhibitions. The studio Fuse*Factory, a firm based in Modena with expertise in the field of digital technologies and design, was appointed to design the exhibition. This, as from the brief provided by the museum architect and the future curator, was supposed to be inspired by the main exhibition of the *Museo Laboratorio della Mente* in Rome (described in the previous chapters) and largely rely on audio-visuals and multimedia installations based on historical records and clinical case histories from the asylum archives. However, the 2008 global financial crisis led to cuts in public funding, which meant the exhibition could not be realised as it was intended (Lanz and Montanari 2022).

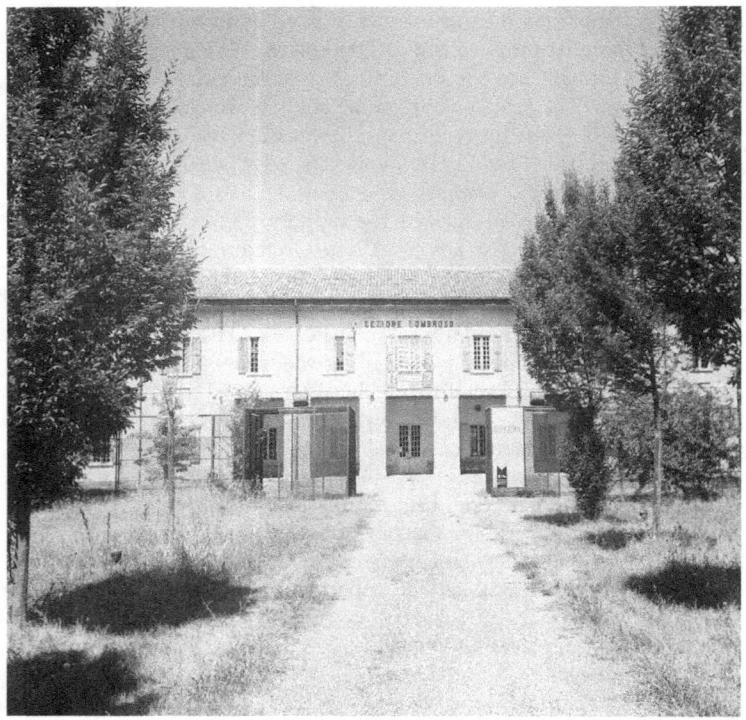

Image 3.2 Former forensic pavilion Lombroso of the former San Lazzaro asylum in Reggio Emilia, now *Museo di Storia della Psichiatria*.
Photo by Francesca Lanz, July 2021.

The *Museo di Storia della Psichiatria* opened in 2013 with the primary mission of serving as a place displaying the history of the San Lazzaro hospital and promoting knowledge and awareness about mental health care in the past and the present (Grassi et al. 2013; Tagliabue 2013). The museum holds a rich archive – comprising the original asylum archives, which includes about 100,000 medical records, a photographic collection of over 1,500 pictures and 1,000 boxes of various administrative documents of different kinds – conserved at the *Biblioteca Scientifica Carlo Livi,* together with the former asylum's bibliographic collection and a diverse collection of objects.[4] The latter dates back to 1875, when it was first established by the asylum superintendent doctor Carlo Livi and then expanded in the following years by his successors. It includes medical objects, objects related to the life and material culture of the asylum and a collection of over 28,000 artworks including drawings, paintings and small terracotta objects. The collection was exhibited for the first time in 1980, in the temporary exhibition titled *Il Cerchio del Contagio* [*Chain of Infection*] (Bergomi 1980) and then conserved by the *Biblioteca Scientifica Carlo Livi*. The former asylum museum collection and 8,000 artworks are today on display at the *Museo di Storia della Psichiatria*. A visitable archive, a gallery for patients' artworks and a workshop room are located at the upper level; the main exhibition is on the ground floor, set up in the spaces that once were the pavilion refectory, the inmates' cells and the yard.

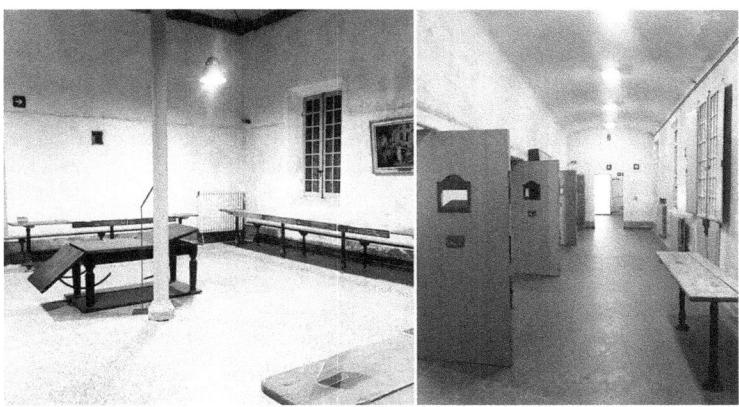

Image 3.3 Museo di Storia della Psichiatria, Reggio Emilia, Lombroso pavilion, former San Lazzaro Asylum.
On the left: The first museum room set up in the old refectory. On the right: The former cells restored and used as exhibition spaces. Photo by Francesca Lanz, December 2019.

During our first interview, when discussing the museum exhibition and its project, Chiara Bombardieri remarked on how the selection of objects to be displayed has been a matter of great thought with the imperative aims of avoiding slipping into morbid voyeurism and challenging stereotypical beliefs of the asylum solely as a place of torture and disrepair (Grassi et al. 2013; Tagliabue 2013).[5] A limited number of objects were eventually selected to be included in the main exhibition together with an audiovisual installation presenting the personal stories of some patients hospitalised at San Lazzaro and, crucially, the former Lombroso pavilion itself. Objects on display all relate to the different therapies used during the working life of the hospital. These include some iconic pieces, such as a 20th-century containment bed and straitjacket, a few pre-19th-century mechanical restraint tools and an ECT machine. Most of the objects selected are large and have their own independent visual strength. They are arranged freestanding in the space, usually with no cases and just a simple square plinth when needed. The display is accompanied by a rather botched informative apparatus consisting of short labels for each object, providing only its denomination and date, very dense panels with text and images and some hand-outs. These are meant to support self-guided tours, but these are, in effect, strongly discouraged in favour of the free guided tours offered by the museum for the general public on weekends and for schools on weekdays.[6]

A guided visit lasts about two hours for the public and three for schools, and it is led by a museum guide flanked by a 'cultural mediator'. The latter is an 'expert by experience', i.e., a person who has experienced mental health problems and is now in a recovery phase. Their involvement in the museum activity is part of their recovery project, but also a key element in the visit. Cultural mediators accompany every guided tour, reading aloud selected excerpts from historical clinical records and some texts written by contemporary patients of the local mental health support services. For school visits, a workshop with cultural mediators is included as part of the visit experience: this is a one-hour, face-to-face, on-site meeting, during which the cultural mediators share their lived experience, respond to students' questions, and talking with them about mental health. The guided tours for the public and for schools differ slightly in their format but share the core feature of the visit to the main exhibition lead by a museum guide. Each visit follows a protocol designed by the museum curator, Chiara Bombardieri, which is adapted by each museum guide, building on their own knowledge of the place, their personal reaction to and interaction with the site and those of past and current visitors.[7] The tour, using Andrea Witcomb's term, can be described as a 'pedagogy of walking' (Golding 2017; Witcomb 2012). The visit structure unfolds around the objects on display, the space's architectural and material elements to narrate the story of the hospital and to prompt questions and discussion with and among the visitors around some key topics.[8] As Cecilia Rodéhn discusses in her article on educational practices in a mind museum, the '"pedagogy of walking" involves a multitude of emotions that encourage visitors to feel' (Rodéhn 2020: 204) and this is especially the case of a guided tour offered at the *Museum of Medical History* in Uppsala described by Rodéhn, which is very similar to the one implemented in Reggio Emilia. As I could also experience and as confirmed by the museum guides during our interviews, empathetic engagement is both as a goal of the tour and an emotional status that characterises the way it is conducted, not only for visitors but also for the guides themselves.

After welcoming visitors in the front yard, the visit starts in the old canteen. Here the guide stands in front of two painting hinged on walls: a reproduction of 1795 painting Dr. *Philippe Pinel at the Salpêtrière*, by

Tony Robert-Fleury depicting Pinel ordering the removal of chains from patients at the Paris asylum for insane women, and a paint of a bird-eye view of the San Lazzaro Asylum in the early 20th century. The guide gives a brief historical introduction about the advent of and within the moral treatment in asylums and San Lazzaro's origins and development. After that, visitors are invited to gather around two objects positioned at the centre of the space and guess without too much thinking what these object are and which was their use. The objects are two 19th-century wooden chairs, called the Guicciardi chairs, invented and realised at the San Lazzaro for physiotherapy and muscles rehabilitation; however, most visitors at first instinctively misunderstand them as torture chairs or electric chairs. This misunderstanding is used by the guide to trigger curiosity and at the same time to challenge the visitors' visual stereotypes about what an asylum was. Visitors' attention is then turned towards the table and benches arranged along the walls and firmly fixed on the floor of the room, which was the former canteen, to discuss about control and how this was enforced in the asylum and in this pavilion particularly as it was the forensic ward of the asylum. From here, the visit continues in the next room, the cells, the yard and the second floor with the object stores and the patients' artwork gallery. As Boyd and Huges note, 'a museum encounter is not a simple matter of being acted upon, but it involves a multitude of enactments of rhythms, tones, affects, and sensations which themselves produce effects' (Boyd and Huges: 6). The rest of this chapter will explore visitors' encounters with the *Museo di Storia della Psichiatria* as they are remembered by visitors and with key regards to their impact and effect on them.

I carried out fieldwork and visitor in Reggio Emilia from December 2020 to July 2021. This involved archival research, interviews with museum staff and architects, and silent participation to various guided tours for the general public (5) and schools (2), observing visitors behaviour in the museum. All that was eventually complemented by two sets of qualitative interviews with museum visitors.[9] The first consisted of 13 remote individual unstructured photo- or video-elicited narrative interviews, for a total of over 11 hours of recordings. Participants were recruited online – mainly via Facebook – with the help of the museum, museum guides and the civic museum network of Reggio Emilia. Some responded voluntarily; others were contacted directly by me. The only requisite for taking part in the study was having visited the *Museo di Storia della Psichiatria* at least once; participants in the study visited the museum from 8 months up to 8 years before the interview.[10] The second set of interviews consisted of four semi-structured in-person and onsite group interviews with nine research participants in total. While the first series of interviews focused on participants' memories of the visiting experience, the second worked as a limitus test recording visitors' reactions and impressions in the heat of the moment. During the online interviews, I started by asking my participants when they visited the museum, how and· with whom and then I posed to them one single and very open question: *Potresti raccontarmi la tua visita al museo, come la ricordi?* [Could you please recount me your visit as you remember it?] This part of the interview was followed by some questions picking up from their account of the visit and revolving around the question: *Che cosa ti ha colpito durante la visita al museo?* [What struck you during your visit?]

The second part of the interview was photo elicited. I asked my participant to look at the pictures together [*guardare insieme le foto*]. Looking at pictures together is something you do after a holiday; and you usually do it with friends to share memories of a nice experience. To me, it was not only a way to revive memories, compare the imagined and remember with the actual and visual, but also a way to create a connection with my participants. It was also way to elicit emotions and prompt reflections associated with their encounter with the museums and to create a space for conversation. Each participant had also been asked before the interview to select up to five images from their visit, if they had any, and to send them to me by email a few days before the interview. I asked them to select those images they considered more relevant and meaningful. I gave them a quite open brief for selecting the images, asking for 'pictures of *something that they consider important* in the museum, or emblematic; pictures of something linked with *something they had seen, heard or felt* during the visit; or pictures of *something that caught their attention* when they visited and that does or does not still resonate in their memory today'. However, I was open to the possibility that these images could simply be the only ones taken during the visit or the only picture still available today in their archives; that was fine, too. During the interview, participants could choose in which order they wanted to look at the pictures. Questions I asked them were: Can you tell me more about this image? Do you remember when and why you took this picture? Why did you select it? What emotions did it elicit in you today? I also asked if there were pictures they thought they took but they could not find in their archive. Or if there were pictures, they would like to have taken but they didn't because sometimes the unphotographed is as telling as what was photographed. When participants did not have any picture to share, I resorted to elicitation using a video of the museum realised by a professional studio for the museum.[11]

Memory anchors and 'emphatic unsettlements'

As with previous studies on museum visitors' memories (Falk and Dierking 2013), my study at the Reggio Emilia museum found that the museum experience generated long-term memories. All the participants declared they could 'remember extremely vividly' their visit, even when it happened a long time ago, and the majority of them did. Virtually all of them remembered a great deal of their visit, with no or very few gaps; the structure of their reports were consistent with the actual structure of the visit protocol, the contents they could remember were often quite accurate; several of them were able to recollect detailed information quite precisely and with little effort. During the analysis of the interviews, I noted how participants' accounts of the visit tended to become more vivid, emotionally engaged and densely clustered around some specific objects and spaces. John Falk and Lynn Dierking make a similar observation about their visitor studies. In their book, *The Museum Experience Revisited,* they note that participants 'anchored their recollections in memories of the physical context' (2013: 206). The authors then discuss how, although they depend on each visitor's personal and sociocultural context, these anchoring points are usually concrete elements of the museum, being either part of its architecture, exhibition design or display, that help people recollect their visit by locating its contents in time and space, and connecting the visit experience with the 'feel and gestalt of the museum' (*ibid.,*: 209). Similarly, in my study, I observed the role of certain elements in fixing the museum experience in people's memories of their visit and helping its recollection. Usually these elements were also the subjects of the selected images. I called these elements 'memory anchors.' These are museum objects, spaces and architectural details and interpretative materials that may or may not be at the centre of the museum project, but that endure in visitors' memories of their visit experience.

Having asked research participants to select up to five images of their visit, it was to be expected that such elements depicted in the pictures would have played a key role in the recollection of the visit. Not least because first, during the visit, they caught the participant's attention and were thus photographed; then, because the pictures of such objects have been selected as significant and emblematic of that visit for it to be recounted; and finally, because they have been the subject of specific attention and discussion during the photo-elicited interview. However it shall be emphasised that these objects had not been photographed within a planned visitor studies workshop, but such photos were spontaneously taken by each visitor during their visit with no other intent than to visually record their visit. When they took them they did not know that these objects and pictures would be used within an interview to recount their experience; rather participants *a posteriori* selected them as reminders to be used as the basis for discussing with me what they encountered at the museum. During the photo-elicited part of the interview, these images eased the recollection of the visit recollection by anchoring memories, as in Falk and Dierking, but also, crucially, they were prompts for broader conversations and reflections. It became clear during the interviews that these objects and spaces not only fixed and recalled memories of the visit, but unlatched emotions associated with it. Looking at these images with me encouraged them to elaborate reflections starting from such emotions, and this was done in most cases spontaneously or with minimum encouragement from me. In doing so, the participants always made connections between the past and the present, between what they encountered at the museum and their own foreknowledge and experiences, often at a very personal level. For it is a generally accepted assumption that the construction and re-construction of memories of a visit are key to how people make meaning out of their visiting experience (Crane 1997), it follows that these elements are key not only in understanding how people remember their visit but also in assessing its impact on them.

The idea of a memory anchor, as I deploy it here, does not only refer to the role these objects have in 'anchoring' alias fixing, memories of the visit experience into visitors' minds, but also to the degree of free personal interpretation and reflection they allow. In other words, such concept is used here to notably hint at the visitors' connections with these objects and the different and possibly changing 'alignments' they can take with the intended meaning of such objects within the display. This freedom, I argue, is what makes the visit experience not only remembered but long-term, meaningful and impactful. As anyone who can sail may know, it is not only the anchor – i.e. the heavy metal object that is dropped from the boat into the water – that keeps the boat in place, but it is also the chain that connects the anchor to the boat. For an anchoring to work, together with the anchor, the right amount of chain must be lowered in the water: this mainly depends on the depth of the bay, the tide and wind intensity. When the anchor-scope is correctly calculated and the anchoring properly done, it prevents the boat from moving away because the weight of the anchor plus that of the chain together hold it in place, but also because the span of the chain allows the boat some freedom of movement that avoids the anchor dragging. I deploy here the metaphor of the memory anchor to discuss the memories of the museum experience and their implications in the meaning-making process involved in a museum visit, to acknowledge that the chain is as important as the anchor, means stating that the museum device active in the act of remembering and enduring in people's memories is as important as each individual's 'alignment' with it in time.

Although memory anchors are in fact selective and personal, perhaps because of the small size of the Reggio Emilia museum and the few objects on display, some of them were recurrent in partici-pants' pictures and recollections of their visits. This is the case with the *bagno di luce* [the electric light bath] and the Guicciardi chairs. As I noted earlier, the chairs have a key opening role during the guided tour, so it was no surprise that they caught visitors' attention. However, these chairs were central also in the memories of those participants who visited the museum without a guided tour, such as Giuseppe. He visited the museum with a small group, with no guide, during a special opening organised by an independent charity and not by the museum. Giuseppe disliked the museum and remembered little of it, but these objects were the only things of the museum he decided to photograph, and he took more than one picture of them. Furthermore, the motivation he gave me for photographing the chairs was also similar to the one given by other participants for choosing or naming these chairs: they were 'beautiful'. Beauty was an extremely recurrent explanation given by most of the participants when I asked them the reason for taking and selecting a photograph of specific objects. Several mentioned being 'struck by its beauty', others referred to 'the care of the details' and someone else commented on the object 'unharmful' look, the fact that it 'looks like normal', or seemed like 'an everyday object'. More than one used the exact words: 'it is beautiful yet terrifying'. In other words, we may say that the beauty, the care of the design and the familiar look of these objects do not adhere with the common idea in people's imagination of the asylum as a place of pain, mis-care and even torture, and this dis-alignment makes them particularly meaningful and memorable asking for a re-alignment.

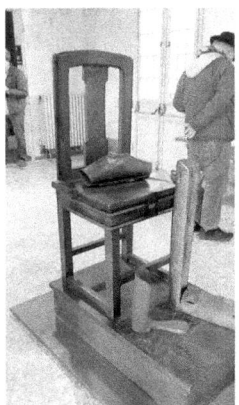 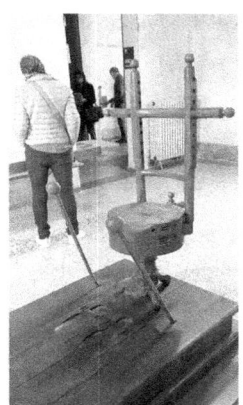 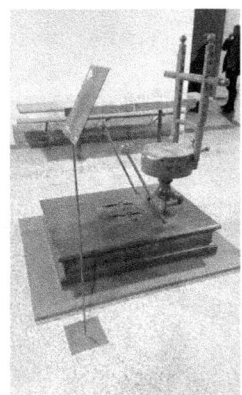

Image 3.4 Museo di Storia della Psichiatria, Reggio Emilia, Lombroso pavilion, former San Lazzaro Asylum.
Photos of the Guicciardi chairs. Photos by Giuseppe Mazzagardi and Elena Montanari (research participants).

Another recurrent memory anchor was the graffiti done in one of patients' cells and representing a map of the territory surrounding Reggio Emilia. The graffiti were featured in many images selected by the participants; they are indeed quite compelling for their visual and emotional power, some of them being quite large works, including drawings and inscriptions carved in the wall plaster. However, the way they endured in people's imagination exceed their visual power. Mattia is a guide at Reggio Emilia civic museums; he is probably the visitor who struggled the most in remembering his visit during our interview. Although he told me he could remember the visit very well, when he started to recount to me his experience, he struggled to do so in a coherent and consistent way and he was quite disappointed with that. He had visited the museum twice – once as a visitor and another one as part of a collaboration between the *Museo di Storia della Psichiatria* and the civic museum where he works – and the memories of the two visits got mixed.[12] Mattia could not find any picture of his visits to the museum, and therefore the second part of our interview was video elicited using an outsourced video. When we were watching the video, Mattia was distracted, disengaged with the interview because he was trying to recollect his memories of the visit that were eluding him. However, when the video arrived in the graffiti cell and these graffiti appeared for a few seconds on the screen, he immediately returned to being focused, active and very engaged. We stopped the video and spent some time on this frame: Mattia was particularly interested in the graffiti depicting a map. He remembered it, although he was sure that the place depicted were named

Image 3.5 Museo di Storia della Psichiatria, Reggio Emilia, Lombroso pavilion, former San Lazzaro Asylum.
Still frame of the video {01:46} in the cell featuring patient's graffiti. Video by Fuse*Factory available on Vimeo https://vimeo.com/222859245 [Last accessed March 2023].

as different local villages, while in fact they are all named Busana. From here we talked about how he felt very lonely and heartbroken thinking about how hard it was for this patient to be far from home, homesick and cut off from his life and his family. We talked about Mattia's sense of belonging to the territory of Reggio Emilia, and after this moment his recollection of the visit started to be more fluid and other memories emerged. For Mattia, as for other participants, memory anchors are such because of their 'familiar' and disturbing nature.

Somehow surprisingly, no one among research participants, expect for one, submitted images of what I previously called 'iconic objects' of mind museums, such as the straitjacket, the ECT or the containment bed. Within a photo-elicited interview, the absence of a picture may be as telling as its presence. One may speculate that because I asked participants to select images of their visit to revive this experience, they might have instinctively refrained from picking images of objects that were emotionally discomforting and could revive uncomfortable feelings. However, some of the objects selected by the research participants were in effect described by them during the interview as 'terrifying', meaning that the search for positive feeling was not a key rationale for taking a picture (or not) nor in selecting it for discussion. Another possible reason for this absence may be related to the fact that such images might be perceived as a stereotype that the participant wants to resist (Rose 2012: 315). This may be the case for such iconic objects of 19th-century psychiatry. Interestingly, the only research participant who selected an image of an iconic object for our interview was Chiara, who works as a mental healthcare professional, and sent me a picture she took at the museum of the straitjacket. When I asked her about this object and the reason for selecting this image, she told me that it compellingly spurred her to think about historic and contemporary types of restraints in mental health care and to question some of her everyday work and standard approaches and practices. The reason Chiara selected the straitjacket is not because it is a broadly symbolic and iconic object of 19th-century psychiatry, nor because of any common visual imaginary related to it, but because for her, it is a 'familiar' object, with which she has a direct and unmediated relationship, one that connected her with the museum. It is not a cliché for her.

As the examples above illustrate, memory anchors are personal and selective. However, there are some commonalities in the reasons they were selected, the way they are remembered and were discussed with me, and the interactions they enable with the museum contents, that provide meaningful insights into what mind museums mean to those who visit them and the impact of such encounter. First, through memory anchors, visitors not only draw connections between the past and the present, but

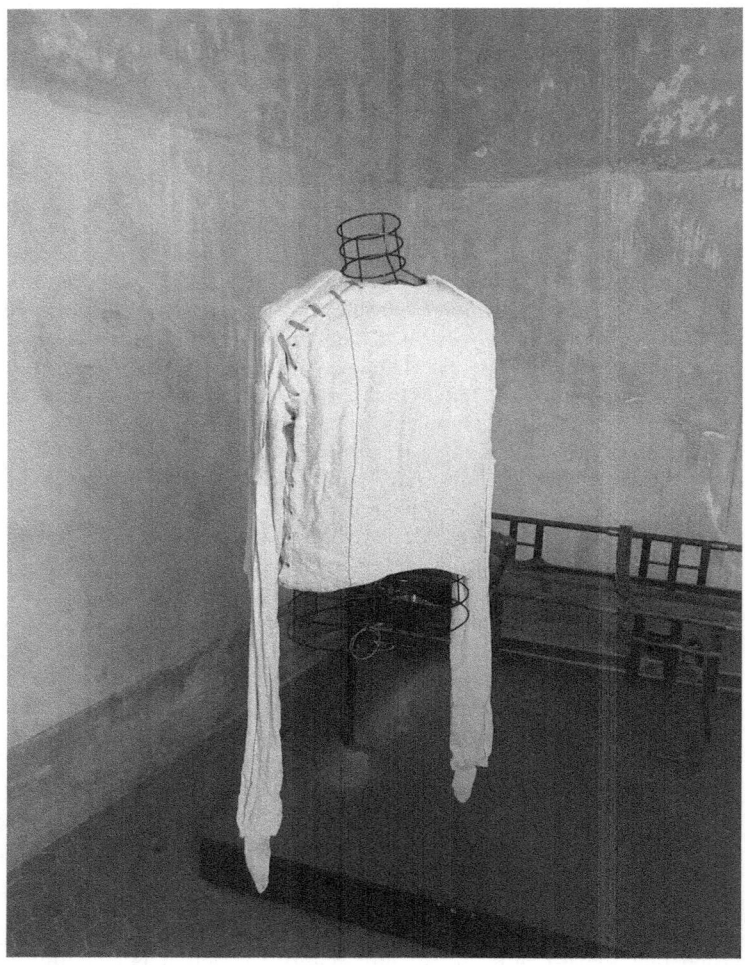

Image 3.6 Museo di Storia della Psichiatria, Reggio Emilia, Lombroso pavilion, former San Lazzaro Asylum.
Photos of the strait jacket display. Photo by Chiara Manfredi (research participants).

they also tend to establish a personal connection with what encountered that not only fixes such objects and the visit experience in their memories, but sustains reflexivity about it afterwards. As mentioned, a key feature of memory anchors is their 'familiar' yet 'challenging' nature. This ambiguity both sparks curiosity and elicits mixed emotions, provoking an emphatic response in the visitors. This backs up what I, with Whitehead, elsewhere argued while discussing the social and political effects of exhibitions hinged on representation of migrants' experience and aimed at eliciting visitors empathetic connection: this is that such affective responses 'may be superficial shows of moral citizenship and an indulgence of momentary sentiment or serious political action, but in either case, the museum helps to legitimise the virtue and, in doing so, to shape an ideal citizenship of empathy for others in a transformation of previous governmental regimes of knowledge of others' (Whitehead and Lanz 2021: 199). When asked about their reasons for visiting the museum, all the participants variously mentioned 'curiosity', which however was not a morbid desire related to visit a place of suffering driven by a sort of voyeurism, but rather a sincere interest in learning more about such places as former asylums were. This is the case, for example, of Elisabetta, Marco, Federica and Giovanna – fictional names – four visitors aged 19 to 21, whom I met on-site. They originate and live in Veneto, a region in the northeast of Italy: they were in Reggio Emilia for a short trip to celebrate Federica's exams, marking the end of high school. When I asked them why they decided to spend a half day visiting this specific museum, they told me that they were curious to see how an asylum was because near their hometown there is an abandoned asylum, they often walk pass it every day, but never could walk inside of it for it is dangerous, and visiting the former San Lazzaro and the museum provided them with the opportunity to learn more about former asylums. For many in Italy, the asylum belongs to the past, but it still resonates in people's lives and memories because of direct connection or by association. For many the asylum may be perceived as a known place for it is indeed are current visual trope in different forms of popular culture although a few ever visited on in real life. The asylum is 'familiar' and yet 'unknown'.

The heritage of mental health, in the form of memory anchors, and in their double nature of common yet disturbing objects, produce a bewilderment in those who encounter them. They do not adhere with visitors' foreknowledge, expectations and imaginaries, and in that visitors' curiosity was reignited. This puts them in a status of attentiveness during their visit, and later sustains reflexivity about what they had encountered. Such re-alignment and its effects are similar to what Susan Crane describes as a positive process of 'distortion' (Crane 1997). 'The "distortion" related to memory and history in the museum' – says Crane – 'is not so much of facts or interpretations, but rather a distortion from the lack of congruity between personal experience and expectation, on the one hand, and the institutional representation of the past on the other' (Crane 1997: 44). Memory is a 'historical process which is frequently interrupted by interpretation to create the present' (*ibid.*). Crane suggests that distortion is not always necessarily equal to a misinterpretation or misappropriation that leads to a misunderstanding; rather, it can create an opportunity space for reflection and 'a means of achieving a constructive, interactive museal experience even in the face of explicit resistance and controversy' (*ibid.,* 50, 57). The analysis of memory anchors in my study support Crane's argument, eventually providing evidence of the positive effect of the museum encounter for visitors in terms of meaning making and potentially supporting my hypothesis about mind museums' capacities to challenge stereotypes about mental health care in the past and support reflections about it in the present.

Finally, what emerged from my study is that visitors experience, encounter and remember mind museums in context. Although the San Lazzaro former asylum has been converted into a public space with public facilities and a public park including several functions unrelated with the museum, visitors look at it differently when they come to visit the museum. All the participants during our interviews did not limit their account to what they saw at the museum but also to the whole area. Many talked, sometimes at length and with several details, about their walk to the museum and back, mentioning other pavilions they passed by, the park, the weather conditions, the light, the temperature and the museum, including its architecture and spaces. Several selected images of the former asylum estate and the exterior spaces. Among the images selected by Chiara for our interview were two of an outdoor space (Image 3.7). She commented: 'I looked at the pavilion name engraved on the façade and I thought how many read it before me and how differently it meant for them.' Chiara, and also other participants, told me how the park and the museum atmosphere encouraged them to think about how these spaces were before: they said that 'in this atmosphere, it was easy to imagine' the past.

This imaginative work enabled them to draw connections between the past and the present, and prompted them to develop introspective and personal reflections. Sometimes this was because of an actual personal direct association with the site – as mentioned, the memory of San Lazzaro still strongly resonates amongst the inhabitants of Reggio Emilia. Francesca (pseudonym) told me about her grandfather, who died at San Lazzaro, after he 'was sent there', having come back from war with syphilis. I met Francesca on-site; she was visiting with a friend, Laura (pseudonym), and after the visit we spent one hour talking about freedom – what it was in the past and what it is in the present and how it is for men and women. Francesca told me she recently divorced, and she asked if her inability to conform to social norms about what a good wife should be would have meant back in time and speculated that she would have been deemed as 'crazy'. However, even those who did not have any direct connection with the site, such as the youngest or people not originating from Reggio Emilia, tended to spontaneously establish a personal connection with the place. Paolo was from Rome. I met him on-site after his visit. He told me that he went for a walk in the park the day before. At the time, he worked as a paramedic on an ambulance for emergency interventions. After his visit during our interview, he was deeply touched by the visit and emotionally upset. During our interview, we spoke for a long time about the lack of assistance given today to families in taking care

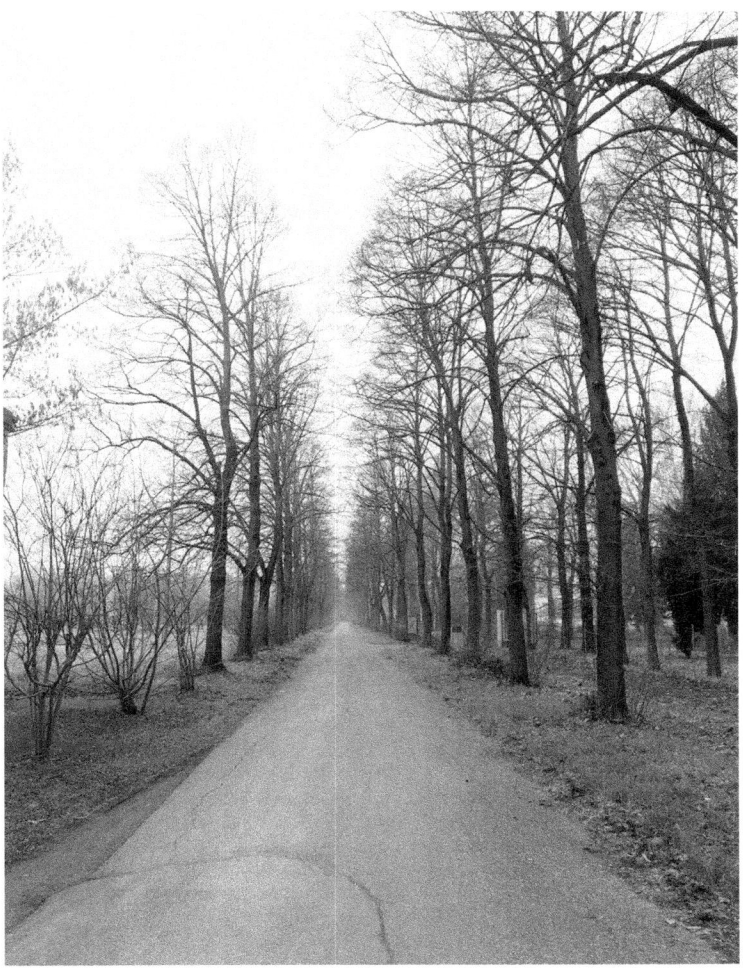

Image 3.7 Former San Lazzaro asylum in Reggio Emilia.
Photos of the lined-tree avenues in the San Lazzaro estate, now a public park.
Photo by Chiara Manfredi (research participant).

of relatives suffering from mental health and he shared with me some personal professional experiences. In such cases, the visit experience begins before entering the museum and continues after it, extending the museum beyond its walls. This observation opens up new questions that scholars have not previously examined pertaining to the agency and cultural relevance of these heritage sites beyond traditional memorialisation practices and that are worth further investigations, which I hope this book will be able to initiate.

Notes

1 This included archival research and a literature review, which encompassed also unpublished and private documents provided to me by the museum curator, Chiara Bombardieri, and the museum architect, Giorgia Lombardini, such as reports, photos, design drawings and personal notes, and a copy of the specialisation thesis by Francesca Gollo, one of the museum guides, including transcripts from three guided tours for high schools.

2 Visual methodologies are increasingly used in qualitative studies and field-work and visitor studies deploying visual methods are rising and becoming popular in museum and heritage studies as well, with promising and interesting results. Among these, the work done by Sumartojo and Graves at the Camps des Milles on materiality, affect and senses at official memory sites is of particular relevance for my study (Sumartojo and Graves 2018; Sumartojo 2019; Sumartojo 2020).

3 Interview with Giorgia Lombardini 4/6/2020.

4 Since the 1980s, the archive and collections of the *San Lazzaro* have been object of several projects aimed at studying, cataloguing them and, most recently, digitalising and making them available online. Medical cases have been catalogued and digitalised as part of the project *Carte da Legare* and can be consulted online at https://cartedalegare.cultura.gov.it/home [Last Accessed, March 2023]. The study of the oldest medical cases conserved in the archive resulted in two scientific monographs, in 2009 and 2011, by Riccardo Panattoni, professor of moral philosophy, and published by Bruno Mondadori (Panattoni 2009). From 2014 to 2017, administrative documents have been catalogued; the two-volume inventory is available online at: https://www.ausl.re.it/Sezione.jsp?idSezione=28833 [Last Accessed, March 2023]. In 2019, a project for the cataloguing and digitalisation of the archive collection began, materials can be accessed through the *IBC* online portal of the *Istituto dei Beni Culturali della Regione Emilia Romagna* (Emilia Romagna Institute for the cultural heritage) and at this link https://bit.ly/3ibPkfJ [Last Accessed, March 2023]. One hundred fifty of the over 28,000 artworks have been objects of a specific study, focussing on *Ars Canusina,* a specific branch of art and craft inspired by Northern Italian Romantic decorative motifs. The collection on display at the *Museo di Storia della Psichiatria* and stored in its visitable archive includes a digital catalogue that can be accessed at: https://bbcc.ibc.regione.emilia-romagna.it/pater/loadcard.do?id_card=26708 [Last Accessed, March 2023].

5 Interview with Chiara Bombardienri 23/12/2019.

6 The museum opening hours are limited to afternoon weekends and prear-ranged school visits on Wednesdays and Thursdays during school terms. However, the museum runs a number of education activities in collaboration with the *Biblioteca Scientifica Carlo Livi,* most of which are targeted at

national high schools with curricula in humanities and social science – with key subjects such as pedagogy, psychology and social anthropology. The museum also runs projects with first and middle schoolchildren with the support of therapists and experts in psychomotion. Occasionally, art projects have also been hosted at the museum, including the multi-award-winning theatrical piece on the painter Ligabue in 2015 by the director Mario Perrotta (http://www.progettoligabue.it/index.php) and a musical project "*La Città del Disordine. Storie di vita dal Manicomio San Lazzaro*" [The City of Chaos. Life Stories from the San Lazzaro Asylum], an album by the musician Nicola Manzan inspired by the study of the historical clinical records of some asylum patients. As part of this project, an audioguide in Italian has been realised in 2022, with the intention to extend opening hours and implement self-guided tours. The audioguide, curated by Georgia Catoni, with text by Chiara Bombardienri and music by Nicola Marzan is available online at: https://www.musei.re.it/collezioni/museo-di-storia-della-psichiatria/audioguide

7 Interview with the museum guides Francesca Poli (20/2/2020 and 7/5/2020), Lucia Romoli (8/5/2020) and Erica Casini (3/6/2020).

8 It is telling how in the online catalogue of the museum collection, the *San Lazzaro* building is listed next to anthropological objects, medical objects and artworks https://bbcc.ibc.regione.emilia-romagna.it/pater/loadcard.do?id_card=26708 [Last Accessed, March 2023].

9 Details about the study are provided in a methodological note included in the Introduction.

10 Among participants in online interviews, the most recent visit was one year before the interview, the more remote eight years before. Although I do not ignore the likelihood that it was people who were more enthusiastic about the museum that stepped forward to participate in the study, the different ways participants have been recruited, the wide participant base and the actual variety of research participants in terms of age, sex, origin and reason for visiting, support the assumption that this group of informants may be considered as a good probability sampling of the museum visitors.

11 *Museo di Storia della Psichiatria*, video by FUSE*FACTORY https://vimeo.com/222859245 [Last Accessed, March 2023].

12 Falk and Dierking (2013) discuss how the different roles we are playing during our visit to a museum change the kind of memories produced by the visit.

Conclusions

The case of the *Museo di Storia della Psichiatria* sets the ground for this concluding reflection pertaining to the 'difficult' nature of the heritage of mental health and its potential to offer a new and productive way to talk about madness today.

First it shall be acknowledged that former asylums are a particularly difficult *built* heritage (Lanz and Montanari 2022). They are linked to a 'past that is recognised as meaningful in the present, but that is also contested and awkward for public reconciliation with a positive and self-affirming identity' and raise questions about their 'public representation and reception,' as well as 'about practices of selection, preservation, cultural comparison and witnessing' (Macdonald 2009: 1). Mental asylums, in fact, have been previously discussed in critical heritage and architectural conservation literature as a 'difficult heritage' (Logan and Reeves 2009), an 'uncomfortable heritage' (Pendlebury et al. 2018), as 'negative places' (Gibbeson 2020) and a 'stigmatized heritage' (Moon et al. 2015). As emerged in the first chapters of this book, built asylums were and are architectural compelxes onto which a great cultural, ideological and political load was and is charged as well as places widely stereotyped and stigmatised in the collective imaginary. Former asylums, are assemblages where different, nested, competing – and sometimes conflicting – identities, memories, meanings, and narratives converge and coalesce within particularly visually powerful, iconic, and evocative physical environments. Because of the specificity of asylum's architecture, the material remnants of former asylums, even when abandoned and neglected, still have the ability today to evoke former uses, acting as a catalyst for sometimes painful memories and emotions. Thus, their mere presence and permanence within our urban landscapes not only can attract curiosity, but also provoke distressing feelings, either at a local community level or on wider scales.

The difficult nature of former asylums historical architectural complexes goes beyond memory issues to involve also designerly considerations. Asylums' specific architectural features in fact make them 'difficult' to reuse from an architectural point of view. Falling within the category of 'uncomfortable heritage', their reuse 'demands not only a change of narrative […] but a very particular negotiation with their architectural built form' (Pendlebury, Wang, and Law 2018: 212), posing dilemmas and hindrances concerning both design and preservation choices and their impact on the meanings and memories associated with the building. Purposely designed around a specific functional and symbolic program, not only do their architectural typology and style inevitably link them to their history of uses and associated difficult memories, but it also makes it very difficult to adapt them to a new function without deeply altering their structure, spaces, and layout (and anyway, in the case of listed buildings, such major transformations may be restricted). Various authors have previously explored the unique challenges of repurposing challenging built heritage for residential, leisure, or third-sector use (Gibbeson 2018; Moon, Kearns, and Alun 2015; Alun, Kearns, and Moon 2013; Alun, Kearns, and Moon 2009; Kearns, Alun, and Moon 2010; Osborne 2003; Franklin 2002a, 2002b). They stress how these interventions involve delicate negotiations, raising questions about strategic forgetting, selective remembrance practices, heritage commodification, and dark tourism (Alun et al. 2013; Pendlebury et al. 2018). Equally, their musealisaton also presents its own set of problems (Lanz and Montanari 2022; Lanz and Whitehead 2019).

Nevertheless, former asylums constitute a European heritage, which although moslty disregarded and often neglected, holds an overlooked potential for disclosing a Europe-wide history, as well as opening a dialogue about urgent current social and cultural issues. My study has proven me that their conservation and valorisation hinges on their reuse, which must be planned and undertaken in a sustainable and relevant way from architectural as well as social and cultural points of view. Such reuse should respect the often-minor, hidden stories embedded and witnessed by these spaces but also allow for its reappropriation and resignification by their new and evolving communities of proximities, including all those individuals or groups who variously today use these sites and/or feel connected to them emotionally. Although I do not ignore nor deny the particularly challenging and awkward nature of such heritage and the dilemmas it raises about its public representation and reception, this study also demonstrates that these buildings, especially when they are converted into cultural public spaces such as mind museums, have a great potential to contribute dismantling stigma by acting as productive everyday places of awareness through 'continual unsettlement', which, as Sharon Macdonald says, is 'what makes these sites potentially so good to think with critically and ethically' (Macdonald 2009: 192).

Second, collections related to asylums and mental health are also themselves a particularly challenging and difficult heritage. As remarked by Catherine Coleborne when discussing, exhibitions on psychiatric history and material culture (Arnold 2005; Coleborne 2001; 2003; 2011; 2020; Coleborne and MacKinnon 2003; 2011a), these collections can prove particularly 'awkward' to exhibit and curate. Many of the objects included in these collections raise difficult ethical dilemmas when displayed in a public exhibition (Veis 2011). Often, their most iconic items, precisely because of their strong visual and imaginative power, risk becoming empty clichés, merely paying lip service to the standard narrative of the horrors of the asylum, where torture overshadowed care. If not handled carefully, the display of these collections may even reinforce stereotypes about mental health and its treatment, contributing to a hardening of views about places and practices of mental health care, both in the past and possibly in the present. Former asylum collections and archives indeed, in fact comply with Macdonald's definition of 'contentious collections', meaning collections that include 'objects and documents gathered up in earlier times according to the scientific ideas, museum ambitions, and opportunities of the days, as well as resulting from the inclinations and even whims of particular curators' (Macdonald 2021: 95). As such, they constitute 'a memory bank' that is today often overlooked and only 'half remembered' (*ibid.,* 96–95). And their display raises disputes and dilemmas about their interpretation and representation, an issue that is also at the centre of mind museum curators' thinking and preoccupations.

Furthermore, as these collections have been, and in many cases still are, somehow hidden, hardly accessible and neglected also, but not solely, for their difficult nature, they have therefore been barely studied (Coleborne and Mackinnon 2011b). The lack of knowledge about contentious collections, notes Macdonald (2021), is one of the underling elements jeopardising their public display. Other considerations complicating and hindering curators' attempts to work with and publicly display these collections and the material heritage of mental health are also related with curators' concerns about 'the voice' of these collections. When looking specifically at former asylums' archives, Coleborne notes, the fact that they 'were *produced about* confined individuals' and within a highly institutionalised setting implies that is very difficult to disentangle these historical textual records from their overall institutional framework and its power dynamics. This, she notes, makes it virtually impossible today to retrieve the genuine patients' voices and lived experiences of care, abuse or institutional violence (Coleborne 2020: 19). Additionally, when working with the materials conserved in these archives, such institutional original nature often creates critical tensions between 'the micro-histories of individual lives, and the overarching narrative of these institutions and their mobile populations' (*ibid.,* 22).

However, as Ken Arnold also remarks '[t]he history of medicine, in theory at last, has a considerable potential to make a profound impact on museum visitors' (Alberti 2011; Arnold 2005: 16; Alberti 2011; Coleborne 2001). Indeed, as the visitor studies carried out at the *Museo di Storia della Psichiatria* also demonstrate, these objects hold a certain power and transformative potential. Because of their somehow familiar look and function, their once intimate physical closeness to the human body, their considerable visual strength and their ability to spark curiosity, they can 'produce responses drawing on profound emotions' (Arnold 2005: 15). Furthermore, examples presented in this book demonostrae how, despite their difficult nature, these collections and former asylums archives today constitute precious resources for the histories of madness, insanity and the asylum. They provide data for the study of patient populations, diagnoses and treatments, as well as insights into their conditions and the asylum life. Their study and critical interpretation can offer the opportunity for re-connecting and re-weaving asylum histories and stories with wider local, national and possibly international social, cultural, political and economic scenarios, with the potential to offer new and unedited perspectives on national histories that may be able to account for mental health and its place in society – a perspective mostly neglected and broadly overlooked in official national historical narratives. The Italian case discussed in this book offers paradigmatic examples of the opportunities offered by these heritage banks.

Finally, another challenge posed by the heritage of mental health concerns its public reception and, in particular how visitors might potentially misunderstand it. However, this preoccupation seems not to find confirmed in the results of my study. Actually, unlike what other authors found in similar studies, especially Dudley in his PhD research on exhibition about mental health (2017; 2018), I did not find any oversimplification nor platitudes in visitor reaction to the exhibition at the Museo di Storia della Psichiatria. Quite the contrary. Even when visitors did not particularly enjoy the museum visit or necessarily 'agree' with the ideas and concept on display, they were moved by such an encounter. What I have found in Reggio Emilia is that the tangible and intangible attributes and characteristics of the museum, its collection and environment actually spur emotional responses and empathic reaction that, in turn, contribute to producing extremely enduring memories in those who visit that sustain personal and introspective reflections. All that, crucially, support responses to the visit experience long after it. All the visitors told me that they had done further research once back home after their visit: reading a book, watching a movie or a documentary, for example. Many of them suggested to other people that they should visit the museum. Some came back with friends – I met several recurrent visitors on-site.

Memory anchors, in particular, demonstrate the potential for mind museums exhibitions to produce what Andrea Witcomb has described as 'emphatic unsettlements' (2012).[1] The material encounter with the heritage of mental health offered by mind museums 'provide access to experience [...] by accessing involuntary memory' (.); the 'surprise' and 'shock' and of this encounter, 'bring the past in tension with present' (*ibid.*, 269) facilitating introspective reflections, producing extremely enduring memories, and prompting proactive reactions to the visit experience. This demonstrates the capability of the heritage of mental health to unlock productive discourses and reflections and possibly contribute to promote awareness about mental health and its care, dismantle stigma and long-lasting stereotypes and offer new ways to 'talk about madness'.

Madness – remarks Andrew Scull – is not a medical term (2011). It is and has always been, however, a matter of medical thinking and investigations that variously interpreted it as an incurable illness, a disease to eradicate, a curable condition, a treatable pathology, an inheritable sickness rooted in the body or a disturbance of the mind determined by socio-affective environmental, conditions and factors. Whilst its impact on our health and wellbeing is all too real and may even extend to causing pain and suffering that can be so deep as to lead to body consumption, unlike other maladies, mental illness can rarely, if ever, be detected by an instrumental medical exam. In very few cases, mental illness can be straightforwardly associated with a causal effect from anomalies in our organs and its evolution hardly ever follows recurrent and predictable prognoses because of the way the sheer variety of different conditions is elusive to examination and largely varies by subjects. Great attention has been devoted in the Western world to the study of the mind and its illnesses across centuries within every culture since ancient Greece and the birth of medicine as a science. The establishment of psychiatry as a specialty within the medical practice at the turn of the 18th century has led in time to the study, experimentation and development of different forms of treatments and approaches to mental health disorders, a large share of which was mostly tentative, often contradictory or in confutation to precedents and today overcome. No different still today, medical treatment of mental illness is an area of medical study particularly rich in uncertainties, unknowns and controversies characterised by an uncommon and deep intertwinement between scientific debate, politics, public opinion and personal experience.

Although 'madness' is not a medical term and despite the fact that it is a word we are all familiar with, today, like many other once-common expressions referring to people's unusual, unconventional, unreasonable and irrational behaviours, it is a largely socially unaccepted term, especially in the context of mental health. The term 'madness' is today considered generalising and particularly stigmatising and offensive or, at the most, provocative and confrontational – as such it is used by many authors in their works on asylums and, in a profoundly different way, by some people who are suffering from mental health issues and who embrace this term as part of their rejection of their psychiatric status and associated treatments.

But 'madness' is more than a term. It is 'something'; something that frightens, fascinates and haunts human imagination; something that disturbs common-sense assumptions, threatens social order, questions institutions and challenges stabilised social practices. Madness plays deep in our consciousness and imaginaries: drawing a line between medical science and evidence and our own imagination and fears might be difficult. An emblematic example of this is the ongoing debate on the therapeutic benefits of ECT mentioned in the second chapter of this book. The very idea of what madness is, how it is understood, managed and perceived has been constantly and considerably changing through time, not only in medical science but also in political discourses, social policies and legislation as well as in philosophical thinking, public opinion and popular culture and beliefs within different geopolitical contexts. Madness has also always been a locus of common clichés and stereotypes in both popular culture and in cultural production, from the more prejudicial and stigmatising ones, to those romantically idealising it as a manifestation of a creative and brilliant mind – 'genius and excess' – proper of an individual gifted with an extraordinary sensibility and innate artistic talents. Madness has long been a trope of artistic production, too, in literature, theatre and visual arts from ancient Greece up to today's film production, including documentaries and successful Hollywood movies, which altogether contributed to shaping collective imaginaries of madness. Since ancient times, madness in the Western world largely and variously tangled with religious beliefs and practices as well as popular superstitions. It had been often associated with demonic possession and supernatural powers, dissolute behaviours and wicked personalities, regarded and treated as a fate or punishment for a lost, sinning soul. Emblematically, the very history of the Bethlem hospital traces back to the 13th century, the Crusades and to a mystic experience in the Holy Land of a Londoner alderman, Simon FitzMary. Nevertheless, madness's very existence, notes Scull, 'has given birth to elaborate sets of social institutions and systems of knowledge that seek to comprehend, to contain, to manage, and to dispose of powerful symbolic and practical challenges madness poses to the social fabric and the very possibility of social order' (2011: 3).

So, what is madness? We may say, with Scull, that madness is a 'common sense category, reflecting our culture's (every culture's?) recognition that Unreason exists' (*ibid.*, 1–2). However, we cannot ignore the fact that, as Foucault put it, what 'reason' and 'unreason' are, is largely a cultural construct and a matter of power and social control. Philosophers and sociologists, as well as psychoanalysts and psychiatrists, have also discussed madness as a social fact and a construct. The works by Foucault himslef and Erving Goffman are the most well-known references of this way of thinking and the antipsychiatric and radical psychiatry movements its on-practice echo. However, albeit no doubt madness was and is a label and a stigma largely determined by place, culture, society, power, gender and class, it is also a 'fact', a brutal reality, which may erupt with anguish in some people's lives at any time and in many different ways, disrupting their certainties, affects, relations and stability. Sometimes it does so abruptly, in a painfully unambiguous and obvious way; other times it happens more subtly and sneakily, yet not less hurtful and unsettling ways. Eventually we shall admit that the possibility to draw a distinction between insanity and normality remains an open and deeply controversial question and the boundaries of madness are, as a matter of fact, ineffable. Perhaps the answer – or better to say the answers – to the conundrum of what is madness, if any and whether they are needed, lie in each and every individual's sensibility. This is the space where the key relevance of mind museums and the heritage of mental health lies.

Note

1 'Essential to [...] them is the ability to not close off the narrative, the requirement that visitors engage imaginatively in the space between themselves and the object or the spatial and esthetic structure of the displays. To do this, visitors require a sense of curiosity, a willingness to engage with a certain opaqueness or to accept that meaning is not reduced to information or instantly available. These exhibitions require emotional and intellectual labor on the part of the visitor through an in-depth engagement with the design of the display, the content, and the physical qualities of the objects/installations. The result is a deeply affective, sensorial form of experience which is palpable while also belonging to the poetic rather than realist or positivist realm. For those who engage with them, they also achieve a movement toward an ethical relationship between ourselves and others in the narratives we tell. The movement is possible because there is a space for us to engage not only with the first-person narratives of what occurred from the point of view of the victim but also to relate this to our own narratives of what happened' (Witcomb 2012: 267).

References

Aglieri Rinella, Tiziano. 2013. "A Cycle of Frescoes: A Narration of Mental Illness at the Museo Laboratorio della Mente in Rome." *IntAR, Interventions and Adaptive Reuse, Difficult Memories: Reconciling Meaning* 4, (April): 59–63.

Ajroldi, Cesare, Maria Antonietta Crippa, Gerardo Doti, Laura Guardamagna, Cettina Lenza, and Maria Luisa Neri (eds.). 2013. *I Complessi Manicomiali in Italia tra Otto e Nocecento*. Milan: Electa.

Alberti, Samuel J. M. 2011. *Morbid Curiosities: Medical Museums in Nineteenth-Century Britain*. Oxford: Oxford University Press.

Allen, Jamie, Jakob Bak, Chris Whitehead, and David Gauthier. 2014. "Seeing Yourself in the Museum: Experimental Actions and Methodological Potentials for Walk-through Studies in Exhibition Contexts." In *Museum Multiplicities: Field Actions and Research by Design*, edited by Luca Basso Peressut, Cristina Federica Colombo, and Gennaro Postiglione, 94–112. Milan: Politecnico di Milano.

Anderson, Jon. 2021. *Understanding Cultural Geography: Places and Traces*. London: Routledge.

Andrews, Jonathan, Asa Briggs, Roy Porter, Penny Tucker, and Keir Waddington. 1998. *The History of Bethlem*. London: Routledge.

Angrisano, Elisabetta. 2019. "L'Ex Ospedale Psichiatrico San Niccolò di Siena: Una Realtà Polimorfa fra Architettura, Archivio e Biblioteca." *Bibliothecae* 8, no. 2: 312–344.

Armiato, Luigi, and Pompeo Martelli (eds.). 2019. "Museo, Memorie e Narrazioni per la salute mentale." *MEFISTO* (special issue) 3, no 2.

Arnold, Ken. 2005. *Cabinets for the Curious: Looking Back at Early English Museums. Perspectives on Collecting*. Aldershot and Burlington: Ashgate.

Babini, Valeria P. 2011. *Liberi Tutti. Manicomi e Psichiatri in Italia: Una Storia del Novecento*. Bologna: Il Mulino.

Bailey, Geoff. 2007. "Time Perspectives, Palimpsests and the Archaeology of Time." *Journal of Anthropological Archaeology* 26, no. 2: 198–223.

Banks, Marcus, and David Zeitlyn. 2015. *Visual Methods in Social Research* (2nd edition). London: Sage.

Barham, Peter. 2020. *Closing the Asylum: The Mental Patient in Modern Society*. London: Process Press.

Barnes, Amy Jane (ed.). 2014. "Forum: Museums and Mental Health." *Museum Worlds: Advances in Research*, no. 2.

Basaglia, Franco (ed.). 1968. *L'Istituzione Negata: Rapporto da un Ospedale Psichiatrico*. Turin: Einaudi.

Baur, Nicole, and Jennifer Melling. 2014. "Dressing and Addressing the Mental Patient: The Uses of Clothing in the Admission, Care and Employment of Residents in English Provincial Mental Hospitals, c. 1860–1960". *Textile History* 45, no. 2: 145–170.

Bennett, Tony. 1998. "The Exhibitionary Complex." *New Formations*, no. 4: 73–102.

Bergomi, Maurizio (ed.). 1980. *Il cerchio del contagio: Il S. Lazzaro tra Lebbra, Povertà e Follia, 1178–1980 (S. Lazzaro: ex padiglione Lombroso, 11–30 aprile 1980)*. Reggio Emilia: Istituti Neuropsichiatrici S. Lazzaro.

Boyd, Candice P., and Rachel Hughes. 2020. *Emotion and the Contemporary Museum: Development of a Geographically-Informed Approach to Visitor Evaluation*. Singapore: Palgrave Macmillan.

Breckner, Ingrid, Massimo Bricocoli, and Corinna Morandi. 2004. "Recinti e Barriere nello Spazio e nella Mente. Riflessioni a Partire dall'Esperienza dell'ex Ospedale Psichiatrico Paolo Pini a Milano." *Territorio*, no. 28: 129–136.

Brooker, Graeme. 2013. "Wastespace." In *Reinventing Architecture and Interiors*, edited by Graham Cairns, 33–52. London: Libri Publishers.

Brooker, Graeme. 2021. *50|50 Words for Reuse – A Manifesto*. London: Canalside Press.

Brooker, Graeme, and Sally Stone. 2004. *Re-Readings*. London: R.I.B.A. Enterprises.

Brooker, Graeme, and Sally Stone. 2019. Re-Readings 2. London: R.I.B.A. Enterprises.

Brookes, Barbara. 2011. "Pictures of People, Pictures of Places: Photography and the Asylum." In *Exhibiting Madness in Museums: Remembering Psychiatry through Collections and Display*, edited by Catharine Coleborne and Dolly MacKinnon, 30–47. New York: Routledge.

Brüggemann, Rolf, and Gisela Schmid-Krebs. 2007. *Verortungen Der Seele – Locating the Soul*. Frankfurt am Main: Mabuse-Verlag GmbH.

Calabria, Verusca. 2020. "The Hidden Memories of Nottingham Mental Healthcare." Research Project funded by National Heritage Lottery Fund. https://www.mentalhealthcarememories.co.uk/ [Last Accessed, March 2023].

Calabria, Verusca, Di Bailey, and Graham Bowpitt. 2021. "'More than Bricks and Mortar': Meaningful Care Practices in the Old State Mental Hospitals." In *Voices in the History of Madness. Mental Health in Historical Perspective*, edited by Robert Ellis, Sarah Kendal, and Steven J. Taylor, 191–215. Cham (Switzerland): Palgrave Macmillan.

Casagrande, Domenico. 2013. "La Follia Reclusa. Alcune Note Critiche sul Museo del Manicomio di San Servolo." *Rivista Sperimentale di Freniatria* CXXXVII, no. 2: 63–73.

Chatterjee, Helen, and Guy Noble. 2013. *Museums, Health and Well-Being*. London: Routledge.

Cherchi, Pier Francesco. 2016. *Typological Shift: Adaptive Reuse of Abandoned Historic Hospitals in Europe*. Syracuse (Italy): LetteraVentidue.

Cirifino, Fabio, Elisa Giardina Papa, and Paolo Rosa. 2011. *Museums as Narration: Interactive Experiences and Multimedia Frescoes*. Cinisello Balsamo (Milan): SilvanaEditoriale.

Cirifino, Fabio, Paolo Rosa, and Leonardo Sangiorgi. 2019. "Musei, Memorie e Narrazioni per la Salute Mentale, Narrazioni, Immagini, Interattività." *MEFISTO* 3, no. 2: 107–120.

Coleborne, Catharine. 2001. "Exhibiting 'Madness': Material Culture and the Asylum." *Health and History* 3, no. 2: 104–117

Coleborne, Catharine. 2003. "Collecting 'Madness': Psychiatric Collections and the Museum in Victroria and Western Australia." In *Madness in Australia: Histories, Heritage and the Asylum*, edited by Catharine Coleborne and Dolly MacKinnon, 183–194. St Lucia, Qld.: University of Queensland Press.

Coleborne, Catharine. 2011. "Collecting Psychiatry's Past: Collectors and Their Collections of Psychiatric Objects in Western Histories." In *Exhibiting Madness in Museums: Remembering Psychiatry through Collections and Display*, edited by Catharine Coleborne and Dolly MacKinnon, 14–29. New York: Routledge.

Coleborne, Catharine. 2020. *Why Talk about Madness? Bringing History into the Conversation*. Cham (Switzerland): Palgrave Macmillan.

Coleborne, Catharine, and Dolly MacKinnon (eds.). 2003. *Madness in Australia: Histories, Heritage and the Asylum*. St Lucia, Qld.: University of Queensland Press.

Coleborne, Catharine, and Dolly MacKinnon (eds.). 2011a. *Exhibiting Madness in Museums: Remembering Psychiatry through Collections and Display*. New York: Routledge.

Coleborne, Catharine, and Dolly MacKinnon (eds.). 2011b. "Seeing and Not Seeing Psychiatry." In *Exhibiting Madness in Museums: Remembering Psychiatry through Collections and Display*, edited by Catharine Coleborne and Dolly MacKinnon, 3–13. New York: Routledge.

Colucci, Silvia. 2007. "Il San Niccolò di Siena da Monastero Francescano a Villaggio Manicomiale: Storia, Architettura e Decorazione (1810–1950)." In *San Niccolò di Siena: Storia di un Villaggio Manicomiale*, edited by Francesca Vannozzi, 79–104. Milano: Mazzotta.

Conolly, John. 1847. *The Construction and Government of Lunatic Asylums and Hospitals for the Insane*. London: John Churchill.

Conolly, John. 1856. *The Treatment of the Insane without Mechanical Restraints*. London: Smith, Elder & Co.

Cooper, David. 1967. *Psychiatry and Anti-psychiatry*. London: Routledge.

Crane, Susan A. 1997. "Memory, Distortion, and History in the Museum." *History and Theory* 36, no. 4: 44–63.

Crippa, Maria Antonietta , and Pier Franco Galliani (eds.). 2013. "Conoscenza, Conservazione, Valorizzazione degli Ex Ospedali Psichiatrici Italiani." *Territorio* 65: 60–105.

Crossley, Nick. 1998. "R. D. Laing and the British Anti-psychiatry Movement: A Socio-Historical Analysis." *Social Science & Medicine* 47, no. 7: 877–889.

Crossley, Nick. 2006. *Contesting Psychiatry: Social Movements in Mental Health*. London: Routledge.

Davis, J. L. n.d. *A History Compiled from Its Annual Reports by J.L Davis, Group Secretary*. UK: Friends of Glenside Hospital Museum.

Deblon, Veronique. 2017. "Constructing the Illusion of Freedom: Architecture and Psychiatry in Nineteenth-Century Belgium." *Journal of Belgian History* XLVII, no. 4: 84–112.

Dernie, David. 2006. *Exhibition Design*. London: Laurence King.

Direzione Generale Archivi. n.d. *Carte da Legare: Archivi della Psichiatria Italiana*. Online portal and thematic section of *SIUSA - Sistema Informativo Unificato per le Soprintendenze Archivistiche* (Italian digital system for archivist superintendencies). https://cartedalegare.cultura.gov.it/home [Last Accessed, March 2023].

Dondici, Damilo. 2009. "Change Minds: Una Storia di Archivi e di Manicomi per Andare oltre la Psichaitria." *MEFISTO* 3, no. 2: 73–83.

Donnelly, Michael. 1992. *The Politics of Mental Health in Italy*. London: Routledge.

Dovey, Kim. 1999. *Framing Places: Mediating Power in Built Form*. London: Routledge.

Drugman, Fredi. 1998. "Architetti per la Scienza. Acrobati Giocolieri Visionari." In *Musei per la Scienza*, edited by L. Basso Peressut. Milan: Lybra Immmagine.

Dudley, Lachlan. 2017. "'I Think I Know a Little Bit about That Anyway, So It's Okay': Museum Visitor Strategies for Disengaging with Confronting Mental Health Material." *Museum & Society* 15, no. 2: 193–216.

Dudley, Lachlan. 2018. "Mental Health in Museums.Exploring the Reactions of Visitors and Community Groups to Mental Health Exhibitions." PhD Diss., Centre for Arts and Social Sciences - Australian National University.

Edensor, Tim. 2005. "The Ghosts of Industrial Ruins: Ordering and Disordering Memory in Excessive Space." *Environment and Planning D: Society and Space* 23, no. 6: 829–849.

Edensor, Tim, and Shanti Sumartojo. 2015. "Designing Atmospheres: Introduction to Special Issue". *Visual Communication* 14, no. 3: 251–265.

Edwards, Rosalind, and Janet Holland. 2013. *What Is Qualitative Interviewing?* London and New York: Bloomsbury.

First Report from the Committee on the State of Madhouses. 1815. London.

Falk, John Howard, and Lynn D. Dierking. 2013. *The Museum Experience Revisited*. New York: Routledge.

Flis, Nathan, and David Wright. 2011. "'A Grave Injustice: The Mental Hospital and Shifting Sites of Memory." In *Exhibiting Madness in Museums: Remembering Psychiatry through Collections and Display*, edited by Catharine Coleborne and Dolly MacKinnon, 101–115. New York: Routledge.

Foot, John. 2014. *La 'Repubblica dei Matti'. Franco Basaglia e la Psichiatria Radicale in Italia, 1961–1978*. Milan: Feltrinelli.

Foote, Kenneth E. 2003. *Shadowed Ground: America's Landscape of Violence and Tragedy*. Austin: University of Texas Press.

Foucault, M. 1961. *Histoire de la folie à l'âge classique - Folie et déraison*. London: Routledge.

Franklin, Bridget. 2002a. "Hospital–Heritage–Home: Reconstructing the Nineteenth Century Lunatic Asylum." *Housing, Theory and Society* 19, no. 3–4: 170–184.

Franklin, Bridget. 2002b. "Monument to Madness: The Rehabilitation of the Victorian Lunatic Asylum." *Journal of Architectural Conservation* 8, no. 3: 24–39.

Fusco, Vera, Francesca Gollo, and Marco Sallustri. 2017. "Reenacting Memories." *FAMagazines* 41, (July–September): 65–71.

Fusco, Vera, Francesca Gollo, and Marco Sallustri. 2019. "Il Museo Laboratorio della Mente come risorsa per la salute Mentale." *MEFISTO* 3, no. 2: 87–106.

Gibbeson, Carolyn. 2018. "After the Asylum: Place, Value and Heritage in the Redevelopment of Historic Former Asylums." PhD Diss., School of Arts and Cultures - Newcastle University (UK).

Gibbeson, Carolyn. 2020. "Place Attachment and Negative Places: A Qualitative Approach to Historic Former Mental Asylums, Stigma and Place-Protectionism." *Journal of Environmental Psychology* 71, no. 8: 1–8.

Gieryn, Thomas F. 2002. "What Buildings Do?" *Theory and Society* 31, no. 1: 35–74.

Goffman, Erving. 1961. *Asylums: Essays on the Condition of the Social Situation of Mental Patients and Other Inmates.* New York, NY: Anchor Books.

Golding, Viv. 2017. "Developing Pedagogies of Human Rights and Social Justice in the Prison Museum." In *The Palgrave Handbook of Prison Tourism*, edited by Jacqueline Z. Wilson, Sarah Hodgkinson, Justin Piché, and Kevin Walby, 989–1010. London: Palgrave Macmillan.

Grassi, Gaddomaria, Elisabetta Farioli, and Chiara Bombardieri. 2013. "Perché Parlare oggi di Psichiatria e della sua Storia: Verso il Museo di Storia della Psichiatria di Reggio Emilia." *Rivista Sperimentale di Freniatria* CXXXVII, no. 2: 75–94.

Griffioen, James. 2009. "Something, Something, Something, Detroit." *Vice.* https://www.vice.com/en/article/ppzb9z/something-something-something-detroit-994-v16n8 [Last Accessed, March 2023].

Guillemain, Hervé. 2013. "I Luoghi della Memoria della Psichiatria Francese." *Rivista Sperimentale di Freniatria* CXXXVII, no. 2: 37–49.

Götz, Aly. 2017. *Zavorre. Storia dell'Aktion T4: L'«Eutanasia» nella Germania Nazista 1939–1945.* Turin: Einaudi.

Harper, Douglas. 2002. "Talking about Pictures: A Case for Photo Elicitation." *Visual Studies* 17, no. 1: 13–26.

Hollis, Edward. 2013. "No Longer and Not Yet." In *Reinventing Architecture and Interiors*, edited by Graeme Cairns, 177–194. London: Libri Publishers.

Hooper-Greenhill, Eilean, and Theo Moussouri. 2001. *Visitors' Interpretive Strategies at Nottingham Castle Museum and Art Gallery.* Leicester: Research Centre for Museums and Galleries.

Jay, Mike. 2016. *This Way Madness Lies: The Asylum and Beyond.* London: Thames and Hudson

Joseph, Alun, Robin Kearns, and Graham Moon. 2009. "Recycling Former Psychiatric Hospitals in New Zealand: Echoes of Deinstitutionalisation and Restructuring." *Health & Place* 15, no. 1: 79–87.

Joseph, Alun, Robin Kearns, and Graham Moon. 2013. "Re-Imagining Psychiatric Asylum Spaces through Residential Redevelopment: Strategic Forgetting and Selective Remembrance." *Housing Studies* 28, no. 1: 135–153.

Kartch, Falon. 2017. "Narrative Interviewing." In *The SAGE Encyclopedia of Communication Research Methods*, edited by Mike Allen. Thousand Oaks: SAGE.

Kearns, Robin, Alun Joseph, and Graham Moon. 2010. "Memorialisation and Remembrance: On Strategic Forgetting and the Metamorphosis of Psychiatric Asylums into Sites for Tertiary Educational Provision." *Social & Cultural Geography* 11, no. 8: 731–749.

Kearns, Robin, Alun Joseph, and Graham Moon. 2012. "Traces of the New Zealand Psychiatric Hospital: Unpacking the Place of Stigma." *New Zealand Geographer* 68, no. 3: 175–186.

Keene, Danya E., and Mark B. Padilla. 2014. "Spatial Stigma and Health Inequality." *Critical Public Health* 24, no. 4: 392–404.

Krznaric, Roman. 2016. *Empathy: Why It Matters, and How to Get It*. London: Random House.

Labrum, Bronwyn. 2011. "'Always Distinguishable from Outsiders': Materialising Cultures of Clothing from Psychiatric Institutions." In *Exhibiting Madness in Museums: Remembering Psychiatry through Collections and Display*, edited by Catharine Coleborne and Dolly MacKinnon, 65–83. New York: Routledge.

Lanz, Francesca 2012. "CityMuseums in Transition: A European Overview." In *European Museums in the 21st Century*, edited by Luca Basso Peressut, Francesca Lanz, and Gennaro Postiglione, 409–485. Milano: Politecnico di Milano.

Lanz, Francesca. 2014. "CityMuseum in a Transcultural Europe." In *Museums and Migration: History, Memory and Politics*, edited by Laurence Gourievidis, 27–43. London: Routledge.

Lanz, Francesca. 2020. "Reusing Atmospheres, the Case of the Adaptive Reuse of the Lombroso Pavilion." In *Ambiances, Alloæsthesia: Senses, Inventions, Worlds*, edited by Damien Masson, 150–155. International Ambiances Network.

Lanz, Francesca. 2021. "The Adaptive Reuse of Neglected Buildings." In *Contested Spaces, Concerted Projects*, edited by Cristina F. Colombo and Jacopo Leveratto, 68–85. Siracusa: LetteraVentidue.

Lanz, Francesca. 2023. "The Building as a Palimpsest: Heritage, Memory and Adaptive Reuse Beyond Intervention." *Journal of Cultural Heritage Management and Sustainable Development*.

Lanz, Francesca, and Christopher Whitehead. 2019. "Exhibiting Voids." In *Handbook of Art and Global Migration*, edited by Burcu Dogramaci and Birgit Mersmann, 331–348. Berlin and Boston: De Gruyter.

Lanz, Francesca, and Elena Montanari. 2022. "The 'Museumization' of Difficult Built Heritages and the Role of Digital Technologies." In *Museum Media (ting): Emerging Technologies and Difficult Heritage*, edited by Theopisti Stylianou-Lambert, Antigone Heraclidou, and Alexandra Bounia, 175–198. New York and Oxford: Berghahn Books.

Lanz, Francesca, and Jacopo Leveratto. 2023. "Exhibitions and Interior Architecture: What Exhibition Design Do?" In *Visiting the Art Museum: A Journey through Disciplines*, edited by Eleonora Redaelli, 67–87. Cham (Switzerland): Palgrave Macmillan.

Law, John. 2004. *After Method: Mess in Social Science Research*. London: Routledge.

Leiknes, Kari Ann, Lindy Jarosh-von Schweder, and Bjørg Høie. 2012. "Contemporary Use and Practice of Electroconvulsive Therapy Worldwide." *Brain and Behavior* 2, no. 3: 283–344.

Lenza, Concetta. 2023. "I Complessi Manicomiali in Italia: Problemi Storiografici e Prosepttive di Valorizzazione." *Territorio* 65: 62–67.

Lindauer, Margaret. 2006. "The Critical Museum Visitor." In *New Museum Theory and Practice: An Introduction*, edited by Janet Marstine, 203–225. Oxford: Blackwell.

Littlefield, David, and Saskia Lewis. 2007. *Architectural Voices: Listening to Old Buildings*. Hoboken, NJ: Wiley.

Lloyd, Justine, and Linda Steele (eds.). 2022. "Special Issue on Critical Perspectives on Sites of Conscience." *Space and Culture* 25, no. 2.

Logan, William, and Keir Reeves. 2009. *Places of Pain and Shame: Dealing with 'Difficult Heritage'*. London: Routledge.

Lombardini, Giorgia. n.d. *I Lavori di Recupero del Padiglione Lombroso all'interno del P.R.U. San Lazzaro*. Project Reports with photographic material, unpublished. Comune di Reggio Emilia, Area Ingegneria e Gestione delle Infrastrutture.

Luciani, Domenico (ed.). 1999. *Per un Atlante degli Ospedali Psichiatrici Pubblici in Italia*. Fondazione Benetton Studie e Ricerche.

MacKinnon, Dolly. 2011. "Snatches of Music, Flickering Images and the Smell of Leather: The Material Culture of Recreational Pastimes in Psychiatric Collections in Scotland and Australia." In *Exhibiting Madness in Museums: Remembering Psychiatry through Collections and Display*, edited by Catharine Coleborne and Dolly MacKinnon, 84–100. New York: Routledge.

Macdonald, Sharon. 2005. "Enchantment and Its Dilemmas: The Museum as a Ritual Site." In *Science, Magic and Religion: The Ritual Process of Museum Magic*, edited by Mary Bouquet and Nuno Porto, 209–227. New York and Oxford: Berghahn Books.

Macdonald, Sharon. 2006. "Words in Stone?: Agency and Identity in a Nazi Landscape." *Journal of Material Culture* 11, no. 1–2: 105–126.

Macdonald, Sharon. 2009. *Difficult Heritage*. New York: Routledge.

Macdonald, Sharon. 2021. "Contentious Collections, Contentious Heritage. Risks and Potentials of Opening Europe's Memory Bank." In *Contentious Cultural Heritage and the Arts: A Critical Companion*, edited by Marion Hamm and Klaus Schönberger, 95–127. Klagenfurt/Celovec: Wieser Verlag.

Machado, Rodolfo. 1976. "Old Buildings as Palimpsest: Towards a Theory of Remodelling." *Progressive Architecture* 11: 46–49.

MacLeod, Suzanne, Laura Hourston Hanks, and Jonathan Hale (eds.). 2012. *Museum Making: Narratives, Architectures, Exhibitions*. London: Routledge.

Maj, Barnaba. 2013. "'Museen der Seele'. Prospettive di Teoria della Storiografia." *Rivista Sperimentale di Freniatria* CXXXVII, no. 2: 15–29.

Mandelli, Elisa. 2019. "Lo Sguardo e la Performance. Le Relazioni tra Medico, Paziente Psichiatrico e Spettatore dal Cinema Medical al Museo Multimediale." *MEFISTO* 3, no 2: 121–134.

Martelli, Pompeo, Claudia Demichelis, Marco Salustri, Gianna Capannollo, and Vera Fusco. 2013. "Contro l'Invisibilità un Museo di Narrazione: Il Museo Laboratorio della Mente." *Rivista Sperimentale di Freniatria* CXXXVII, no. 2: 51–62.

Martelli, Pompeo. 2019. "Una Nuova Introduzione 10 Anni Dopo." In *Museo Laboratorio della Mente and Studio Azzurro*, edited by Museo Laboratorio della Mente and Studio Azzurro. Cinisello Balsamo: Silvana Editoriale.

Mason, Rhiannon, Areti Galani, Katherine Lloyd, and Joanne Sayner. 2018a. "Experiencing Mixed Emotions in the Museum: Empathy, Affect, and Memory in Visitors' Responses to Histories of Migration." In *Emotion, Affective Practices, and the Past in the Present*, edited by Laurajane Smith, Margaret Wetherell, and Gary Campbell, 124–148. Abingdon: Routledge.

Mason, Rhiannon, Alistair Robinson, and Emma Coffield. 2018b. *Museum and Galleries Studies: The Basics*. London: Routledge.

McLaughlan, Rebecca. 2015. "Corrupting the Asylum: The Diminishing Role of the Architect in the Design of Curative Environments for Mental Illness in New Zealand." *Architectural Theory Review* 20, no. 2: 180–201.

Miller, Daniel. 2005. "Materiality: An Introduction." In *Materiality*, edited by Daniel Miller, 1–50. Durham (US): Duke University Press.

Miorandi, Paolo. 2022. *Nannetti: La Polvere delle Parole*. Rome: Exorma

Moon, Graham, Robin Kearns, and Alun Joseph. 2006. "Selling the Private Asylum: Therapeutic Landscapes and the (Re)Valorization of Confinement in the Era of Community Care." *Transactions of the Institute of British Geographers* 31, no. 2: 131–149.

Moon, Graham, Robin Kearns, and Alun Joseph. 2015. *The Afterlives of the Psychiatric Asylum: The Recycling of Concepts, Sites and Memories*. Burlington and Farnham: Ashgate.

Museo Laboratorio della Mente and Studio Azzurro (eds.). 2019. *Museo Laboratorio della Mente*. Cinisello Balsamo: Silvana Editoriale.

Moser, Stephanie. 2010. "The Devil is in the Detail: Museum Displays and the Creation of Knowledge." *Museum Anthropology* 33: 22–32.

Osborne, Ray. 2003. "Asylums as Cultural Heritage: The Challenges of Adaptive Re-Use." In *'Madness' in Australia: Histories, Heritage, and the Asylum*, edited by Catherine Coleborne and Dolly MacKinnon, 217–230. St Lucia, Qld.: University of Queensland Press.

Panattoni, Riccardo. 2009. *Lo Sguardo Psichiatrico: Studi e Materiali dalle Cartelle Cliniche tra Otto e Novecento*. Milan: Mondadori.

Pancheri, Paolo, and Maria Caredda. 1999. "L'ECT nella Schizofrenia." In *Trattato Italiano di Psichiatria*, edited by Paolo Pancheri and Giovanni Battista Cassano, 1750–1757. Milan: Masson.

Pascarelli, Pietro (ed.). 2013. *Rivista Sperimental di Freniatria* (Special Issue) CXXXVII, no. 2.

Paulson, George W. 2012. *Closing the Asylums: Causes and Consequences of the Deinstitutionalization Movement*. Jefferson, North Carolina: McFarland & Co.

Pendlebury, John, Yi-Wen Wang, and Andrew Law. 2018. "Re-Using 'Uncomfortable Heritage': The Case of the 1933 Building, Shanghai." *International Journal of Heritage Studies* 24, no. 3: 211–229.

Philo, Christopher. 2004. *A Geographical History of Institutional Provision for the Insane from Medieval Times to the 1860's in England and Wales*. Lewiston (UK): Edwin Mellen.

Piddock, Susan. 2003. "The 'Ideal Asylum' and Nineteenth-Century Lunatic Asylums in South Australia." In *Madness in Australia: Histories, Heritage and the Asylum*, edited by Catharine Coleborne and Dolly MacKinnon, 37–48. St Lucia, Qld.: University of Queensland Press.

Piddock, Susan. 2007. *A Space of Their Own: The Archaeology of Nineteenth Century Lunatic Asylums in Britain, South Australia and Tasmania*. New York: Springer.

Pink, Sarah. 2006. *The Future of Visual Anthropology: Engaging the Senses*. Abingdon: Routledge.

Pink, Sarah. 2013. *Doing Visual Ethnography*. Los Angeles and London: SAGE.

Pink, Sarah. 2015. "Going Forward Through the World: Thinking Theoretically About First Person Perspective Digital Ethnography". *Integrative Psychological and Behavioral Science*, 49, no. 2: 239–252.

Pink, Sarah. 2020. "A Multisensory Approach to Visual Methods." In *The SAGE Handbook of Visual Research Methods*, edited by Luc Pauwels and Dawn Mannay, Chapter 33. Los Angeles and London: SAGE.

Pink, Sarah, and Shanti Sumartojo. 2018. *Atmospheres and the Experiential World*. London: Routledge.

Pink, Sarah, Shanti Sumartojo, Deborah Lupton, and Christine Heyes LaBond. 2017. "Empathetic Technologies: Digital Materiality and Video Ethnography." *Visual Studies* 32, no. 4: 371–381.

Plevoets, Bie, and Koenraad Van Cleempoel. 2019. *Adaptive Reuse of the Built Heritage: Concepts and Cases of an Emerging Discipline*. London: Routledge.

Porter, Roy. 2002. *Madness: A Brief History*. Oxford: Oxford University Press.

Proctor, Robert N. 1988. *Racial Hygiene: Medicine under the Nazis*. Cambridge, MA: Harvard College.

Robert, Phillippe. 1989. *Adaptions: New Uses for Old Buildings*. Princeton: Architectural Press.

Rodéhn, Cecilia. 2020. "Emotions in the Museum of Medical History. An Investigation of How Museum Educators Employ Emotions and What These Emotions Do." *International Journal of Heritage Studies* 26, no. 2: 201–213.

Rondinone, Troy. 2019. *Nightmare Factories: The Asylum in the American Imagination*. Baltimore: Johns Hopkins University Press.

Roppola, Tiina. 2012. *Designing for the Museum Visitor Experience*. London: Routledge.

Rose, Gillian. 2012. *Visual Methodologies: An Introduction to Researching with Visual Materials*. London: SAGE.

Scull, Andrew (ed.). 1981. *Madhouses, Mad-Doctors, and Madmen: The Social History of Psychiatry in the Victorian Era*. Philadelphia: University of Pennsylvania Press.

Scull, Andrew. 2011. *Madness: A Very Short Introduction*. Oxford, USA: Oxford University Press.

Ševčenko, Liz. 2010. "Sites of Conscience: New Approaches to Conflicted Memory." *Museum International* 62, no. 1–2: 20–25.

Ševčenko, Liz. 2011. "Sites of Conscience: Heritage of and for Human Rights." In *Heritage, Memory and Identity*, edited by Helmut Anheier and Yudhishthir Raj Isar, 114–123. London: SAGE.

Sienaert, Pascal, and Walter Van den Broek. 2009. "Electroconvulsive Therapy in Continental Western Europe: A Literature Review." In *Electroconvulsive and Neuromodulation Therapies*, edited by Conrad M. Swartz, 246–255. Cambridge: Cambridge University Press.

Silverman, Lois H. 2002. "The Therapeutic Potential of Museums as Pathways to Inclusion." In *Museums, Society, Inequality*, edited by Richard Sandell, 69–83. London and New York: Routledge.

Smith, Laurajane. 2021. *Emotional Heritage: Visitor Engagement at Museums and Heritage Sites*. London: Routledge.

Smith, Laurajane, Margaret Wetherell, and Gary Campbell (eds.). 2018. *Emotion, Affective Practices, and the Past in the Present*. Abingdon: Routledge.

Smith, Leonard. 2017. "Lunatic Asylum in the Workhouse: St Peter's Hospital, Bristol, 1698–1861." *Medical History* 61, no. 2: 225–245.

Stastny, Peter, and Darby Penney. 2008. *The Lives They Left Behind: Suitcases from a State Hospital Attic*. New York: Bellevue Literary Press.

Stevenson, Christine. 2000. *Medicine and Magnificence: British Hospital and Asylum Architecture, 1660–1815*. Yale: Yale University Press.

Stylianou-Lambert, Theopisti, Alexandra Bounia, and Antigone Heraclidou (eds.). 2022. *Emerging Technologies and Museums: Mediating Difficult Heritage.* New York and Oxford: Berghahn Books.

Sumartojo, Shanti. 2016. "Commemorative Atmospheres: Memorial Sites, Collective Events and the Experience of National Identity." *Transactions of the Institute of British Geographers* 41, no. 4: 541–553.

Sumartojo, Shanti. 2019. "Sensory Impact: Memory, Affect and Sensory Ethnography at Official Memory Sites." In *Doing Memory Research*, edited by D. Drozdzewski and C. Birdsall, 21–37. Singapore: Palgrave Macmillan.

Sumartojo, Shanti. 2020. "New Geographies of commemoration". *Progress in Human Geography*, 45, no. 3: 531–547.

Sumartojo, Shanti, and Matthew Graves. 2018. "Rust and Dust: Materiality and the Feel of Memory at Camp des Milles." *Journal of Material Culture* 23, no. 3: 328–343.

Sumartojo, Shanti, and Pink Sarah. 2018. *Atmospheres and the Experiential World.* London: Routledge.

Tagliabue, Luigi. 2013. "Il valore di un Museo della Psichiatria a Reggio Emilia." *Rivista Sperimentale di Freniatria* CXXXVII, no. 2: 95–111.

Taylor, Jeremy. 1981. *Hospital and Asylum Architecture in England, 1840–1914: Building for Health Care.* London: Mansell

Topp, Leslie, James Moran, and Jonothan Andrews (eds.). 2007. *Madness, Architecture and the Built Environment.* London: Routledge.

Tuke, Samuel. 1813. *Description of the Retreat, an Institution near York for insane persons of the Society of Friends containing an account of its origins and progress, the modes of treatment and a statement of cases.* Historical resource avaialbe on welcome trust online repository. https://wellcomecollection.org/works/dcy3yd8x

Tzortzi, Kali. 2015. *Museum Space: Where Architecture Meets Museology.* Farnham: Ashgate.

UN - United Nations. 1991. *Principles for the Protection of Persons with Mental Illness and the Improvement of Mental Health Care. Principles for the Protection of Persons with Mental Illness and the Improvement of Mental Health Care.* Adopted 17 December 1991 by General Assembly resolution 46/119.

UOS Centro Studi e Ricerche ASL Roma and Studio Azzurro. (eds.). 2012. *Museo Laboratorio della MentePortatori di Storie Da Vicino Nessuno è Normale.* Cinisello Balsamo: Silvana Editoriale.

2019. *Unhinged: On Jitterbugs, Melancholics and Mad-Doctors.* Ghent: Hannibal.

Valentini, Valentina (ed.). 2017. *Studio Azzurro: L'Esperienza delle Immagini.* Milan and Udine: Mimesis.

Veis, Nurin. 2011. "The Ethics of Exhibiting Psychiatric Material." In *Exhibiting Madness in Museums: Remembering Psychiatry through Collections and Display*, edited by Catharine Coleborne and Dolly MacKinnon, 48–61. New York: Routledge.

Watson, Sheila. 2015. "Emotions in the History Museum." In *The International Handbooks of Museum Studies: Museum and Theory*, edited by Andrea Witcomb and Kyle Message, 259–484. Chichester: Wiley-Blackwell.

Whitehead, Christopher. 2016a. *Why Analyze Museum Display?* https://eprints.ncl.ac.uk/223873 [Last Accessed, October 2021].

Whitehead, Christopher. 2016b. *How to Analyze Museum Display: Script, Text, Narrative.* https://eprints.ncl.ac.uk/237369 [Last Accessed, October 2021].

Whitehead, Christopher, and Francesca Lanz. 2020. "'Only Connect': The Heritage and Emotional Politics of Showcasing the Suffering Migrant." In *Connecting Museums*, edited by di Mark O'Neill e Glen Hooper, 186–202. London: Routledge.

Witcomb, Andrea. 2012. "Understanding the Role of Affect in Producing a Critical Pedagogy for History Museums." *Museum Management and Curatorship* 28, no. 3: 255–271.

Yanni, Carla. 2007. *The Architecture of Madness: Insane Asylums in the United States.* Minneapolis: University of Minnesota Press.

Index

abuse 11, 25, 29, 31, 34, 108
accumulation 36, 52
acquisitions 48, 68
advocacy 1
After Methods (Law) 84–5
Alberti, Samuel 41
Alzheimer, Alois 23
amateur museums 48
Anderson, Jon 5, 36
Andrews, Jonathan 39
anthropological criminology 37n7
antipsychiatry 5, 25–6, 56, 67
antipsychotic drugs 25
architectural/architecture 16–17, 21,
    106–7; history 9, 15; typology
    14, 16, 107
Arnold, Ken 109
art therapy 63–4, 80n6
art workshop 80, 80n6
asylum museums 4, 46–56, 65–8, 70,
    83; birth of 47; collections
    in 108
asylums 3, 20, 24; architecture 16–17,
    21, 106–7; archives 45, 90, 108;
    before asylum 9–13; building
    1; collections 40–1, 46, 108;
    complexes 16; curative ability
    of 22–3; description of 8–9;
    development 9; forensic ward
    of 93; geography and
    architectural histories of
    15–16; as heritage 2; histories
    50, 109; hospital admissions to
    43; imagination of 97–8;
    influences on local
    development 21; inmates 43;
    institutions 57–8; management
    and maintenance 42; material

culture 47; medical and social
    rationale of 16; memorabilia
    52; memories and memorabilia
    of 50; origins and harbingers
    of 12; palimpsests 29–36;
    pavilions 88; personal
    memorabilia of 50; planning
    and design of 14; popular
    culture of 53–4; population 22;
    proximity of 28, 30; rise and
    development of 12; rise and
    fall of 21–9; rooms and spaces
    of 57; spaces and ambiances
    53; unique buildings 14–21;
    visual culture of 54; in
    Western Europe 8–9;
    see also asylum museums
attachment, consequence of 52
audio recording 72

Baccei, Enza 63–4, 81n17
Bailey, Geoff 36
Basaglia, Franco 5, 26, 38n11
Basaglia Law 57
Baur, Nicole 43
Beckenham community 78
behaviours 12–13, 17, 20, 25, 37, 43,
    93, 110–11
Belgium asylum 14, 56
Bennett, Tony 39–40
Benthamite panopticon model 15
Bethlem asylum 10, 39, 60, 73
Bethlem Museum of the Mind 60, 66,
    73, 75, 77–8
Bethlem Royal Hospital in Beckenham
    56, 61
Biblioteca Scientifica Carlo Livi 42,
    89–91

For Product Safety Concerns and Information please contact our EU
representative GPSR@taylorandfrancis.com
Taylor & Francis Verlag GmbH, Kaufingerstraße 24, 80331 München, Germany